PocketGuide to Treatment in Occupational Therapy

PocketGuide to Treatment in Occupational Therapy

Franklin Stein, Ph.D., OTR/L

Department of Occupational Therapy
University of South Dakota
Vermillion, South Dakota

Becky Roose, M.S., OTR/L

Medilink Services, Inc.
Des Moines, Iowa

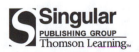

Singular
PUBLISHING GROUP
Thomson Learning™

Singular Publishing Group
Thomson Learning
401 West A Street, Suite 325
San Diego, California 92101-7904

> **Singular Publishing Group, Inc.,** publishes textbooks, clinical manu-
> als, clinical reference books, journals, videos, and multimedia materials
> on speech-language pathology, audiology, otorhinolaryngology, special
> education, early childhood, aging, occupational therapy, physical ther-
> apy, rehabilitation, counseling, mental health, and voice. For your
> convenience, our entire catalog can be accessed on our website at
> *http://www. singpub.com*. Our mission to provide you with materials to
> meet the daily challenges of the ever-changing health care/educational
> environment will remain on course if we are in touch with you. In that
> spirit, we welcome your feedback on our products. Please telephone **(1-
> 800-521-8545)**, fax **(1-800-774-8398)**, or e-mail (*singpub@singpub.com*)
> your comments and requests to us.

© 2000, by Singular Publishing Group

Typeset in 9/11 Stemple Schneider by Black Dot Group
Printed in Canada by Transcontinental Printing

Library of Congress Cataloging-in-Publication Data

Stein, Franklin.
    Pocket guide to treatment in occupational therapy / by Franklin
Stein, Becky Roose.
      p.   cm.
    Includes bibliographical references.
    ISBN 0-7693-0025-1 (softcover : alk. paper)
    1. Occupational therapy Handbooks, manuals, etc.   I. Roose,
Becky. II. Title.
    [DNLM: 1. Occupational Therapy Handbooks. WB 39 S819p 2000]
    RM735.3.S74 2000
    615.8'515—dc21
DNLM/DLC   98-36125
for Library of Congress   CIP

ABBREVIATED CONTENTS

Preface

The main purpose of this PocketGuide is to enable students and clinicians to have a quick reference for planning treatment strategies. The treatment suggestions are pragmatic and are meant to be user friendly. They can serve as an initial step in planning treatment. However, good treatment is evidence based, supported by clinical research. The treatment suggestions are based on the authors' clinical experiences, research, and extensive reading. In using this PocketGuide, it is important that the reader understand what is good treatment:

1. It is individually planned to meet the needs and interests of the client. This implies that the therapist in conjunction with the client plan a treatment strategy that is client-centered and collaborative and is in synch with the treatment team.
2. Treatment should be holistic, taking into consideration the biopsychosocial factors that impact on function. For example the hand therapist also considers the psychological and social aspects of a client's disability, and the psychosocial occupational therapist considers the client's physical functions.
3. Treatment is based on an experimental design where the client is assessed before and after intervention. This implies that the therapist will establish a baseline of function, implement the treatment strategy, and then reassess function.
4. The treatment method should be operationally defined so that the strategies can be easily identified and replicated by other therapists. Treatment protocols can be established by the therapist and individualized to meet the needs of the client. Treatment should not be a cookbook formula, yet there should be structure and guidelines.

5. The effects of the treatment should be continuously reevaluated by the therapist, client, family, teacher, and interested others to determine whether the treatment should be continued, changed, or discontinued.
6. Treatment in general should be eclectic, meaning that the frames of reference or theories generating treatment are selected to meet the functional goals of the client. For example psychodynamic, cognitive-behavioral, occupational performance, and developmental frames of reference can all be applied to the same client.
7. Treatment should be evidence-based and supported by research findings. Good treatment can be substantiated by explaining to the client how and why the treatment works.

How the PocketGuide is Organized

Basically the PocketGuide is organized around the major disabilities that occupational therapists encounter in their every day practice. These include physical, psychosocial, geriatric, and pediatric diagnoses. Treatment guidelines are outlined for the major disabilities. In addition there are brief descriptions of the treatment techniques that therapists use and definitions of terms that are relevant to treatment such as abduction and positive symptoms.

Each main entry is printed in bold and blue color. Each cross-referenced entry is underlined in blue. Each main entry disorder is listed alphabetically, with subcategories of a given disorder described under the main entry.

Specific techniques, most applicable across disorders, also are alphabetized and described at their main alphabet entry. When appropriate, the reader is also referred to the disorders for which the technique is appropriate.

The appendixes include an outline of muscles and movements, drawings of major splints, orthotic devices, and web addresses of health organizations, tables of muscles, average range of motion measurements, prime movers for upper and selected lower extremity motions, and substitutions for muscle contractions.

Abduction.   See <u>Anatomical position</u>.

Active Assistive Range of Motion (A/AROM).   See <u>Range of motion</u>.

Active Range of Motion (AROM).   See <u>Range of motion</u>.

Activities of Daily Living (ADLs).   Tasks that are essential for self-care, including dressing, grooming, feeding, mobility/transferring, bathing, and toileting. See <u>Self-care</u>, <u>Assistive technology</u>, and specific diagnoses/conditions for further discussion and treatment.

Activity Analysis.   A process of evaluating the steps and components involved in an activity. When a patient works toward goals, appropriate activities should be used to improve the patient's impaired functions. Various activities can address multiple performance components while the patient completes one task. For example, a patient who places rings on a ring tree can be improving AROM, muscle strength, right or left awareness, compensation for visual field cuts, coordination, position in space, or proprioception. The analysis of an activity not only assists the therapist in choosing activities to address multiple goals simultaneously, but it also prevents the therapist from using an activity that does not work toward the patient's goals. The activity analysis is also a detailed examination of a task into performance components such as sensorimotor, cognitive, and psychosocial factors. The significance and meaning of a task to an individual is considered as well as the sequential steps necessary in completing a task. When activities are used in treatment, the therapist considers the interests of the client, cultural factors, and the abilities of the client to complete the activity. The therapist embeds the treatment goal, such as increasing grip strength or stress management, into the task and relates it to a performance area such as <u>Work</u>, <u>Leisure</u>, and <u>Self-care</u>. The activity should be age appropriate and gradable so that the therapist can modify it and adapt it as the client improves.

Activity Group Therapy. Originally developed by Samuel Slavson (1943) for treating children with behavior disorders. Slavson advocated a permissive environment where children act out their impulses through play and behavioral interactions. The goal of therapy is to help the child develop inner controls in an unstructured and free environment. Creative media such as clay, fingerpaints, water colors, and blocks can be used to help children express themselves nonverbally.

Acupuncture. An ancient Chinese treatment technique that is based on the concept of a vital energy flow or life force (ch'i) which is thought to circulate through the body along meridians similar to the blood vessels or neural circuits. Practitioners of acupuncture insert needles into identified meridians of the body to relieve pain. Some scientists explain that the effectiveness of acupuncture is that endorphins (opiates) are released when a needle is placed in the meridian point. Acupuncture is also being used in a number of illnesses such as drug addiction and asthma. Research results have been encouraging.

Adaptation. The adjustment of a person to his or her environment as a reaction to a stressor or environmental demand. For example a therapist can help an individual with arthritis by adapting eating utensils with build-up handles for easier grasp. Adaptation also refers to the modification of an environment (e.g., wheelchair ramps, self-care equipment, or assistive technology to enable the individual to function independently in <u>Work</u>, <u>Leisure</u>, or <u>Self-care</u>).

Adaptive Equipment. Devices that have been adapted to help a patient complete a <u>Self-care</u>, <u>Work</u>, or <u>Leisure</u> activity with increased independence. See <u>Assistive technology</u> for further discussion and applications during treatment.

Adaptive Skills. Newly learned behavior that helps the individual to be independent in performance areas, such as

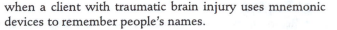
when a client with traumatic brain injury uses mnemonic devices to remember people's names.

Adduction. See Anatomical position.

Adhesions. Fibers that connect two tissues that are not normally connected. Therapists often use this term when referring to scars and scar tissue which forms in collagen "clumps," and can adhere a structure such as a tendon to the underlying bone or overlying skin. See Hand injuries for further discussion and treatment.

Treatment
* Special scar pads which provide pressure to the scar may help reduce adhesions.
* The patient can also be taught to use Friction massage to keep structures from adhering to one another.

Adult Day Care. Supervised social, recreational, and health related services for clients who have cognitive, emotional and physical impairments. Individuals with Alzheimer's disease can benefit from day care. Caregivers can also benefit from the respite that allows them to continue their activities during the day and to work.

Aerobic Exercise. Repetitive movements of major muscle groups while the body utilizes large amounts of oxygen that is transported through the arteries, as in walking, running, dancing, biking, and swimming. It has been shown to be an effective activity in treating Depression, Anxiety, and cardiovascular disorders. Most health professionals recommend that normal individuals should engage in at least moderate exercise for 30 minutes every day to maintain a healthy cardiovascular system.

Affect. The mood of an individual such as depressed, angry, happy, manic, anxious, relaxed, fearful, elated, or hostile. Disorders of affect include Depression and manic-depression. Treatment for affect or mood disorders includes Prescriptive exercise, creative expression, Stress management, Relaxation therapy, and Biofeedback.

Flat Affect
- Refers to dull, unresponsive emotions where the client has difficulty expressing feelings.

After-care Clinic. A state or locally funded agency that is an extension of the state or county hospital designed to provide a transition to the community. Services provided can include case management, supervision of medication, counseling and psychotherapy, vocational placement, and occupational therapy. Individuals with chronic mental illness and substance abuse can benefit from this service.

Agnosia. Inability to interpret sensory information. See Cognitive-perceptual deficits for treatment.

Agonist. A muscle that completes a desired motion. For example, if the desired motion is elbow flexion, the agonist is the biceps (along with the brachialis and brachioradialis). The agonist may also be referred to as the Prime mover.

Agraphesthesia. The inability to identify letters, numbers, or symbols that are traced on the skin while vision is blocked. See Cognitive-perceptual deficits for treatment of perceptual deficits.

Agraphia. The inability to write.

Airplane Splint. A splint used to prevent limitations in shoulder abduction ROM. The patient's upper extremity is usually positioned near 90° of shoulder and horizontal abduction. Patients who have had burns and skin grafts of the upper extremity will benefit from this splint. See Splints for further examples of splints and their application to particular diagnoses.

Akinesia. Difficulty with the initiation of voluntary movement. This deficit results from a lesion in the basal ganglia. Patients who have Parkinson's disease may display akinesia. See Parkinson's Disease for treatment and further discussion.

Alexander Technique.   A body technique, developed by
an Australian actor in the 1890s, to correct the posture of
the head, neck, and spine by bringing the way we move
under our conscious direction and avoiding a buildup of
muscular tension. It involves balance and movement therapy used to improve postural habits currently causing
fatigue. The therapist, who is certified in this technique,
helps the client to develop natural and painless movement
patterns through hands-on guidance. The therapist observes the client's breathing patterns, movements, and posture while the client walks, stands and sits, and bends over.
Recommendations are made to the client to incorporate
healthy movement patterns into his or her everyday Work
and Leisure. Anecdotal evidence claims that it is effective in
relieving tension headaches, neck and back pain, and muscle spasms. It may be potentially useful for clients who
have had a stroke, multiple sclerosis, and other neurological
diseases.

Alexia.   The inability to read.

Alzheimer's Disease.   A chronic, progressive disorder
that most often occurs in people over 65 years old. It is
accompanied by a degeneration of the cerebral cortex and
other areas of the brain, which results in impairment of cognitive functions. The cause is unknown. It is characterized
by memory loss, personality deterioration, confusion, disorganization, language distortions, sleep and eating disturbances, and difficulties with Self-care functions. Individuals
with Alzheimer's disease can benefit from music programs,
sensory stimulation, outdoor walking, arts and crafts, and
pet therapy.

Specific Treatments
- Complete exercises to maintain range of motion and
  mobility
- Utilize gross motor activities for exercise and leisure
  when fine motor activities become difficult

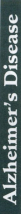

- Fabricate splints to prevent contractures or deformity if weak antagonist muscles are unable to oppose strong agonist muscles
- Maintain balance through reaching activities
- Teach compensation techniques for memory loss such as a daily written schedule, notebook, calendar, list, or map
- Give simple directions for tasks to increase the patient's ability to follow verbal commands
- Provide orientation to person, place, time, and situation with a written orientation board or other tool
- Increase or maintain the patient's self-esteem through the performance of Self-care and Leisure activities
- Implement the use of routines, schedules, and organized environments to increase the patient's independence with activities and reduce anxiety/fear
- Complete community outings or involve the patient in group therapy/support groups for socialization

Contraindications/Precautions

- The patient is at risk for becoming lost, even in a familiar environment such as the nursing home or neighborhood
- Give the patient realistic expectations regarding the prognosis of the disease and the goals of treatments; do not instill a sense of false hope
- Avoid environments that may be overstimulating; organize treatment areas to reduce distractions
- Monitor the patient's safety judgment when responding to dangerous situations such as a hot stove or a smoke alarm
- If a splint has been fabricated, monitor for skin breakdown or decreased circulation
- Avoid the use of sharp objects if the patient is in the final stage of Alzheimer's disease

Americans with Disability Act (ADA) of 1990 (CPB-101-336). Refers to the civil rights of individuals with disabilities. It is organized into 5 titles. Title I, Employment, insures that an individual with a disability who can perform a job with or without reasonable accommodation cannot be discriminated against. Title II, Government nondiscrimination, insures that individuals with disabilities will have the necessary transportation and access to federal, state, and local public services. Title III, Private business, refers to public accommodations and services operated in the private sector. Title IV, Telecommunication, insures that individuals with speech and hearing impairments have reasonable accommodation from telephone companies to facilitate communication. Title V refers to complaint procedures and miscellaneous items such as access to federal wilderness areas.

Amputation. Removal of all or part of an extremity that can occur spontaneously from a trauma or surgically to remove a diseased part of the body. For example, a patient who has diabetes may have sores that will not heal and contain infection; amputation may be required to prevent spread of infection. Amputation may also be indicated for a patient who has peripheral vascular disease. Amputation is completed at a level on the extremity where the physician feels good wound-healing and proper fit for prosthetics can occur.

Specific Treatments
- Following surgery, teach the patient to don and doff the prosthesis
- Allow the patient to use the prosthesis functionally during activities; if upper extremity amputation has occurred, treatment should begin with the prosthetic extremity assisting the unaffected extremity and progress to use of the extremity in one-handed activities
- Instruct the patient to use the unaffected limb to compensate for motor or sensory loss in the affected limb; for example, the patient should learn to test the temperature of bath water with the left hand, even though the patient may have always used the right hand for this activity in the past

- Teach the patient proper care and maintenance of the prosthesis
- Desensitize the stump of the affected extremity if the patient is hypersensitive and has difficulty wearing the prosthesis
- Discuss the emotional adjustment to the loss of the extremity
- Encourage the patient to join a support group or complete activities for socialization
- Train specific skills required for return to work or leisure activities as needed
- Explore new interests and aptitudes if the patient is unable to return to the previous work or leisure activities
- Educate the patient on assistive devices that can assist with self-care or transfer activities
- Complete a home evaluation and recommend adaptations to the environment as needed for the patient's safety and mobility after return home

Contraindications/Precautions
- Teach the patient to inspect the skin of the stump to check for breakdown from use of the prosthesis
- Monitor the prosthesis to ensure that it works correctly

Amyotrophic Lateral Sclerosis.   A nervous system disorder that affects the upper and lower motor neurons and various tracts of the spinal cord. This disease results in weakness and atrophy of all voluntary muscles except those that control the eye and sphincters. Upper motor neuron involvement results in spasticity and decreased strength, while lower motor neuron involvement results in flaccidity and muscle atrophy. Onset is frequently between the ages of 35–65 years of age. The cause is unknown. Symptoms often begin distally and asymmetrically, with many patients first noticing weakness in the hands. Upper motor neuron involvement and spasticity occur later in the disease process. Other symptoms include muscle fasciculations, especially in the extremities and tongue; dysphagia; dysarthria; hyperactive deep tendon reflexes; and difficulty with breathing. Death usually occurs from respiratory failure 2–5 years after onset of the disease.

Specific Treatments

- Fabricate splints to maintain functional positions in the presence of weak muscles
- Recommend assistive devices as needed to continue the completion of functional activities
- Assist the patient with finding a new form of communication, such as a communication board, if Dysarthria hinders language production
- Adjust the patient's diet as needed to reduce chewing or improve swallowing
- Position the patient appropriately, especially during meals for safety in swallowing
- Complete upper extremity exercises to maintain endurance and ROM; aquatic therapy may be particularly useful in this situation
- Teach Pain management techniques
- Educate the patient on Stress management and Relaxation therapy
- Train the patient to complete activities while using energy conservation and work simplification principles
- Instruct the patient on safe and easy transfer methods
- Assist the patient with emotional adjustment to the disease
- Explore new leisure activities which are able to be completed as the disease progresses
- Encourage the patient and family members to join a support group
- Educate the patient on assistive devices which can make Self-care, home management, or transfer activities easier
- If the patient is able to continue working, provide recommendations and/or assist with adaptations to the work environment

Contraindications/Precautions
- Do not have the patient complete resistive exercise as the course of the disease eventually results in weakness, regardless of strengthening activities; instead, focus on exercise to maintain endurance and ROM
- Watch for signs of decreased respiration
- Avoid fatigue
- Monitor the purchase of expensive equipment to keep costs down if possible

Anarithmetria.   Difficulty with math problems that is not due to another reading, writing, or spatial deficit. A patient with this deficit also may have had proper training and demonstrated sufficient academic skills in the past.

Anatomical Position.   When referring to parts of the body, anatomical position is used as the basis for describing parts in relation to one another. The person is standing erect with the head facing forward. The person's upper extremities are alongside the body with the palms facing forward. The person's legs are together with the toes pointing forward (Moore, 1992).

Planes.   Four imaginary planes that pass through the body while it is in anatomical position are used to help with relating body parts to one another.
- **Median Plane:** An imaginary plane that divides the body (or a body part such as the hand or foot) into right and left halves by passing vertically through the body (or body part) from the front to the back.
- **Sagittal Plane:** An imaginary plane that is parallel to the median plane, but does not divide the body into equal halves.
- **Coronal Plane:** An imaginary plane that divides the body into front and back portions by passing vertically through the body from one side to the other. This plane may also be referred to as the frontal plane.

Anatomical Position

- **Horizontal Plane:** An imaginary plane that divides the body into upper and lower portions by passing horizontally through the body from one side to the other.

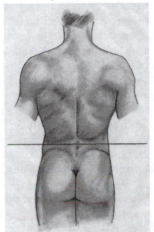

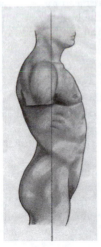

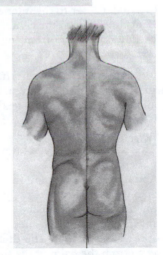

Anatomical Position

Positional adjectives. The use of common adjectives helps describe the relationship of body parts to one another.

- **Superior:** Closer to the person's head. The terms cranial or cephalic may also be used.
- **Inferior:** Closer to the person's feet. The term caudal may also be used.
- **Anterior:** Closer to the front of the body. The term ventral may also be used.
- **Posterior:** Closer to the back of the body. The term dorsal may also be used.
- **Medial:** Closer to the median plane of the body.
- **Lateral:** Farther from the median plane of the body.
- **Proximal:** Closer to the person's trunk or the body part's point of origin.
- **Distal:** Farther from the person's trunk or the body part's point of origin.
- **Superficial:** Closer to the surface of the skin.
- **Deep:** Farther from the surface of the skin.
- **External:** Closer to the exterior surface of a body part.
- **Internal:** Closer to the interior surface of a body part.
- **Central:** Closer to the center of the body or body part.
- **Peripheral:** Farther from the center of the body or body part.

Movement Terms. These terms help describe the movement of a body part at a joint. See Appendix E for specific motions and the normal ranges of those motions.

- **Flexion:** Generally, motion at a joint that bends a body part.
- **Extension:** Generally, motion at a joint that straightens a body part.
- **Abduction:** A joint motion that moves a body part away from the midline of the body in the coronal plane, except when referring to fingers, toes, or the thumb. When the fingers or toes abduct, they move away from the midline of the hand or foot. The thumb abducts when it moves away from the palm of the hand.

- **Adduction:** A joint motion that moves a body part toward the midline of the body in the coronal plane, except when referring to fingers, toes, or the thumb. The fingers and toes adduct when they move toward the midline of the hand or foot. When the thumb adducts, it moves toward the palm of the hand.

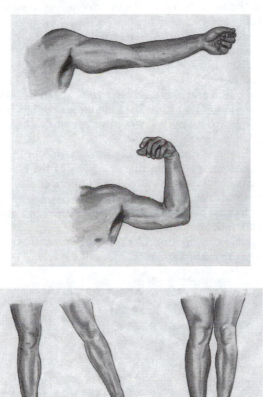

Anatomical Position

- **Horizontal Abduction:** A joint motion at the shoulder that occurs when the shoulder is flexed and results in the arm being pulled away from the midline in the transverse plane.
- **Horizontal Adduction:** A joint motion at the shoulder that occurs when the shoulder is flexed and results in the arm being pulled toward the midline in the transverse plane.
- **Internal Rotation:** Also referred to as medial rotation. A joint motion that turns the anterior surface of a body part medially, or toward the midline of the body, in the transverse plane.
- **External Rotation:** Also referred to as lateral rotation: A joint motion that turns the anterior surface of a body part laterally, or away from the midline of the body, in the transverse plane.
- **Supination:** Rotation of the forearm or foot medially in the coronal plane, so that the palm of the hand or the sole of the foot are facing upward/inward.
- **Pronation:** Rotation of the forearm or foot laterally in the coronal plane so that the palm of the hand or the sole of the foot are facing downward/outward.
- **Inversion:** A motion of the foot that combines supination with adduction of the front of the foot.

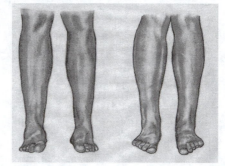

- **Eversion:** A motion of the foot that combines pronation with abduction of the front of the foot.
- **Circumduction:** A joint motion that moves a body part in a circular motion that results from a combination of flexion, extension, abduction, adduction, and rotation.

Ankylosis.   A fixated or stiffened joint often caused by an abnormal bony or fibrous union resulting from a disease process.

Anomia.   See Aphasia.

Anomic Aphasia.   See Aphasia.

Anorexia Nervosa.   An eating disorder that most commonly occurs in females 12 to 21 years old. It is characterized by a fear of being obese and a refusal to maintain normal body weight. The disorder results in emaciation, amenorrhea, body image disturbances, Anxiety, and other emotional reactions. It can be treated by Family therapy, Cognitive-behavioral methods, Prescriptive exercise, Creative arts, Music therapy, Psychoeducational groups, and Stress management. See Bulimia.

Anosognosia.   The inability to perceive that hemiplegia is present following a lesion. See Cognitive-perceptual deficits for further discussion and treatment.

Antagonist.   A muscle that completes the motion opposite to the desired motion. For example, if the desired motion is elbow flexion, then the antagonist to elbow flexion is the triceps, which completes active extension.

Anterior.   See Anatomical Position.

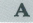

Antisocial Personality Disorder

Antisocial Personality Disorder. Characterized by behaviors such as lying, stealing, aggressiveness, substance abuse, criminal activity, and disregard for authority and discipline. The individual lacks moral and ethical standards, empathy toward others, and is unable to feel guilt. Synonymous terms are sociopathic and psychopathic personality.

Treatment
- Treatment is aimed at helping the individual to develop inner controls and empathy toward others.
- Group treatment has been effective when consensual validation is used to give feedback to the individual.
- Behavior modification has also been successful in changing individuals with severe acting out.

Anxiety. A feeling of apprehension, worry, uneasiness, fear of the future, or dread. Physiological symptoms such as disturbed breathing, increased heart rate, increased sweating, hand tremors, and dizziness frequently accompany anxiety.

Treatment
- Relaxation therapy
- Stress management
- Paradoxical intention
- Systematic desensitization

Anxiety Disorders. Exaggerated fears that prevent or limit an individual from performing normal activities or behavior. They include panic disorders, phobias, stress disorders and obsessive-compulsive behaviors. Physical symptoms often occur with anxiety disorders such as heart palpitations, sweating, hand tremors, chest pain, shortness of breath, dizziness, and nausea.

Treatment
- Behavioral rehearsal
- Systematic desensitization
- Paradoxical intention

16

- Creative arts
- Music therapy
- Stress management
- Relaxation therapy
- Biofeedback

Aphasia.   A language disorder that results from neurological damage, and is often demonstrated by a patient who has had a CVA. A patient with aphasia may have difficulty with expression or comprehension of either written or verbal language. Some patients are affected so profoundly that they are unable to express or comprehend language. Treatment for aphasia includes use of communication boards and cognitive retraining programs.

Types of Aphasia

- **Global Aphasia:** Loss of all language skills, including receptive and expressive ability.
- **Broca's Aphasia:** The inability to express oneself. The patient is able to understand auditory input; however, the patient will demonstrate difficulty with reading, writing, and monetary concepts.
- **Wernicke's Aphasia:** The inability to understand auditory input. The patient is able to express thoughts; however speech is usually rapid and meaningless. The patient may demonstrate the ability to understand single words, but reading and writing complex thoughts will be difficult.
- **Anomia:** Difficulty with word finding that occurs in aphasia. If this is the only deficit demonstrated by a patient, the patient is diagnosed with anomic aphasia.
- **Anomic Aphasia:** A condition characterized by the inability to find words for conversation; however the patient does not demonstrate any other symptoms of aphasia.

Aphonia.   The inability to produce sound from the larynx.

Apraxia.   A perceptual deficit which hinders patients from completing functional or purposeful movement even though the patient demonstrates normal sensory, motor, and coordination skills. See <u>Cognitive-perceptual deficits</u> for further discussion and treatment.

Types of Apraxia

- **Limb Apraxia:** The inability to execute purposeful movements with the limbs, even though the motor and sensory functions of the limb are intact. Limb apraxia can be further subdivided into ideomotor apraxia and ideational apraxia.
  - *Ideational Apraxia:* The inability to complete purposeful movement during functional activities, usually resulting from difficulty with sequencing.
  - *Ideomotor Apraxia:* The inability to complete purposeful movement on verbal command. A patient may be able to complete that same activity spontaneously, but is unable to perform under a testing situation.
- **Constructional Apraxia:** The inability to design or construct pictures, images, or three-dimensional objects. It affects the individual's ability to complete purposeful movements that must occur within a specific spatial relationship or design, specifically writing or constructing dimensional objects.
- **Dressing Apraxia:** The inability to perform movements, which are necessary to complete dressing, even though motor and sensory functions are intact

Approximation.   A compression of joint surfaces that facilitates joint receptors and promotes stability, within the framework of proprioceptive neuromuscular facilitation (PNF) (Voss, 1967, Voss, Ionta, & Myers, 1985). This technique is usually applied during weightbearing as a downward motion through the shoulder, elbow, and/or wrist joints. See <u>Motor control problems</u>, <u>Proprioceptive neuro-muscular facilitation</u> for more techniques.

AROM.   See Active range of motion

Aptitude.   The inherent, natural ability of an individual and the underlying capacity to learn or perform in a specific area. Aptitude tests are used to measure abilities in clerical, mechanical, musical, artistic and computer areas. Occupational therapists use aptitude tests in vocational rehabilitation programs.

Aquatic Therapy.   The therapeutic use of water, hot or cold, fresh or mineral, for the treatment of physical or psychological disorders. An equivalent term is hydrotherapy. The properties of water that contribute to the effectiveness include buoyancy, which decreases a body's weight, surface tension, relative density, viscosity, temperature, and hydrostatic pressure, which increases lung capacity and venous circulation. Therapy with water can be used for decreasing pain, cleansing effects, increasing range of motion and muscle strength, increasing cardiac function, increasing respiratory output, as a diuretic, and to create a relaxing or stimulating psychological effect. Aquatic therapy has also been used successfully in increasing self-esteem and social interactions between the parent and the child. Some of the most common disorders treated with aquatic therapy include orthopedic problems, cerebral palsy, arthritis, multiple sclerosis, TBI, and stroke. There are also definite implications for use with clients experiencing psychosocial disorders.

Aroma Therapy.   The use of essential oils from plants to enhance general health and appearance. There is evidence that oil of lavender and sandalwood are effective in producing a calming effect.

Arousal.   The physiological state of readiness or stimulation of an individual to act, as in Selye's theory of stress (1974), or in the ability to attend to a task.

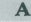

Arthroplasty. Replacement of any or all parts of a joint with manufactured hinges or pieces of bone.

Types of Arthroplasty

Total Hip Arthroplasty. Many surgical approaches may be used. The therapist must communicate with the physician to know the approach used and the necessary precautions. This will ensure that the cement has set and all soft tissue has healed before motions are completed which could displace the manufactured pieces of the joint. Arthroplasty is usually completed in patients who have degenerative joint disease or rheumatoid arthritis. The patient generally must follow precautions for 6–8 weeks following surgery; however, the physician should be consulted to make sure healing is complete before removing the patient's precautions. The patient may be limited to no full weight-bearing on the hip for up to 6 months.

Specific Treatments

- Increase the patient's upper extremity strength to improve the patient's ability to use assistive devices for ambulation
- Complete activities to increase endurance, since any length of hospitalization results in a decrease of activity which may affect endurance
- Teach <u>Pain management</u> or <u>Relaxation therapy</u> if needed
- Instruct the patient regarding safe transfer methods when transferring into a low chair, the bed, the toilet, or the tub
- Educate the patient on hip precautions which may pertain to the patient depending on the approach used during surgery
- Train the patient to use energy conservation and work simplification techniques during activities
- Complete a home evaluation as needed and recommend appropriate equipment to ensure that the patient returns to a safe environment

20

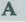

- Instruct the patient on assistive devices that can be used to increase the patient's independence with dressing while observing applicable precautions; devices may include a reacher, dressing stick, sock aid, long-handled shoehorn, elastic shoelaces, or shoe buttons.
- Educate the patient on equipment that may be used to complete bathroom activities independently including grab bars, bath bench, safety frame, and toilet riser.
- Help reorganize the home to prevent the patient from bending, kneeling, or reaching above the head
- Recommend that heavy tasks, such as cleaning and laundry, be completed by others until the patient demonstrates safe ambulation

Contraindications/Precautions

- Instruct the patient to see the physician if infection occurs anywhere in the body, since the site of the hip replacement is at high risk for spread of infection
- Precautions for separate surgical approaches are as follows:
  - Posterior surgical approach
    - → No hip flexion past 80–90°
    - → No hip adduction past midline
    - → No internal rotation of the hip; do not pivot on the affected leg
    - → An abductor pillow should always be placed between the knees when the patient is sidelying
  - Anterior surgical approach
    - → No external rotation of the hip; do not cross the legs
    - → No hip adduction past midline
    - → An abductor pillow should always be placed between the knees when the patient is sidelying
  - Transtrochanteric surgical approach
    - → No hip flexion past 80-90°
    - → No hip adduction past midline
    - → An abductor pillow should always be placed between the knees when the patient is sidelying

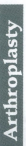

  → No full weight-bearing on the affected leg
  → No internal rotation of the hip
  → No active hip abduction
- Direct lateral surgical approach
  → No hip adduction past midline
  → An abductor pillow should always be placed between the knees when the patient is sidelying
  → No full weight-bearing on the affected leg
  → No active hip abduction
- Communicate closely with physician regarding movement and weight-bearing precautions, since a wrong movement can result in displacement of the joint.

Metacarpophalangeal Joints. Patients who have rheumatoid arthritis often require this intervention.

Treatment

- After the patient has had surgery, he or she should begin gentle active range of motion of the fingers on post-operative days 1–2.
- On days 3–5, the patient may begin gentle active range of motion and active-assisted range of motion of the replaced joint.
- The therapist should teach the patient to complete full fist flexion by first flexing the metacarpophalangeal joints, and then curling the fingers into the palm with proximal and distal interphalangeal joint flexion. If the patient does not learn this technique, he or she may complete full fist flexion by substituting proximal and distal interphalangeal joint flexion for metacarpophalangeal flexion which will lead to stiffness and possible contracture of the replaced joint after a period of time.
- On post-operative days 5–7, the therapist should fabricate a dynamic dorsal splint which holds the affected metacarpophalangeal (MCP) joint in the following position (depending on which joint is affected): index finger MCP = 45° flexion, middle finger MCP = 60° flexion, ring

and small finger MCP = 70° flexion. The patient should wear the splint at all times for 6–8 weeks, except to remove the splint four times a day for 5-minute exercise periods. The patient may begin to use the affected hand with the splint applied during easy functional activities, such as eating, at 2–3 weeks after surgery.

- At 6–8 weeks following surgery, the patient can start mild resistive activities and use the hand for functional activities without the splint applied.

  Proximal Interphalangeal Joints. This arthroplasty may be completed to correct a Boutonnierre or Swan neck deformity. The affected joint may be immobilized with a splint to hold the joint in extension between exercise sessions. The patient may begin gentle active and active-assisted range of motion 2–3 days after surgery. The therapist should support the metacarpophalangeal joint of the affected finger in extension, so that the muscle pull during range of motion exercises directly affects the proximal interphalangeal joint.

Art Therapy. The use of art as a therapeutic tool to provide the opportunity for nonverbal expression, communication, and growth. Art therapy historically was initially influenced by the psychoanalytical movement. One of the important goals of an art therapist is to help the client express one's feeling in a spontaneous manner with the support and encouragement from the therapist. Art therapy is an important modality for individuals who are depressed, anxious, phobic, or are unable to express their feelings verbally. Art therapy is also used with children to help them develop their self-esteem while serving as a perceptual motor activity.

Assertiveness Training. A technique used in behavior therapy to assist individuals with social skills to become more assertive in their interpersonal relationships. Role playing and behavior rehearsal are used in the technique.

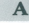

Assistive Technology. Adaptation or creation of a device to assist a person with self-care, work, or leisure activities. The list below provides ideas of equipment that may be helpful in some circumstances; however, this list is by no means exhaustive. Also, a piece of equipment that helps one patient may only confuse another and make the activity more difficult. If possible, a patient should be able to try equipment on a trial basis before purchasing it; this helps ensure that the patient is able to use the equipment successfully. In some instances, the patient may need to try various types of equipment before the best tool is found to promote the patient's independence. Adaptive techniques are also included in the following list, because some devices require special techniques or placement of items.

Self-care activities

Dressing

- Specific garments can be used such as pullover or button-down shirts, sweatpants, elasticized pants, or clothes which are a size larger than usual.
- Brassieres with front closures or sports bras that pull over the head may be purchased. The patient may also be taught to hook a back-fastening bra in the front, and then turn the bra around to the back.
- A dressing stick, which has a small hook on one end and a larger double hook on the other, to help push and pull clothing off and on the extremities.
- A reacher can be used to help with dressing as well as picking items up from the floor if a patient who has a hip replacement is unable to bend past 90°.
- Buttons can be replaced with larger buttons.
- Buttonhooks can assist a patient with hemiplegia in buttoning a shirt with one hand.
- Fasteners can be replaced with Velcro.
- Zipper pulls can be attached to enlarge the pull tab of zippers.

- Elastic shoelaces, shoe buttons, or other shoe devices can allow lace-up shoes to be slipped on or tied with one hand.
- The patient may be asked to purchase Velcro or slip-on shoes to eliminate the need for tying shoes.
- Sock aids can be used with or without garter attachments to help don socks or TED hose. To increase the effectiveness of the sock aid, powder may be used on the patient's foot to promote sliding of the aid on the foot.
- A long-handled or regular length shoehorn will help the patient pull shoes on.

Grooming and Hygiene

- A bath chair or bench allows the patient to transfer into the tub safely by sitting on the edge of the chair first, and then swinging the lower extremities into the tub.
- A hand-held shower will convert a tub only into a shower and prevent a patient from using stairs to use an upstairs or downstairs shower. This also assists the patient with washing the hair.
- A long-handled bath sponge or brush will assist the patient in reaching the lower extremities or back when bathing if the patient has bending precautions or limited ROM.
- A wash mitt aids a patient with weak grasp while bathing.
- Rubber strips can be placed on the bottom of the tub to prevent a patient from slipping.
- Grab bars, which are installed on the wall (in a stud) or fastened to the edge of the tub, increase the patient's ability to stand from the toilet or bath chair.
- An elevated toilet seat prevents a patient with hip precautions from bending past 90°. This device also can assist a patient with standing since it will be easier to stand from a taller device than a short toilet seat.

- A safety frame, which assists the patient with standing and also helps protect the patient who has poor balance from falling, can be placed around the toilet.
- A special device can be used to hold toilet paper and help a patient with toilet hygiene.
- Grooming devices can be adapted with extended or built-up handles to increase independence of a patient with limited ROM or weak grasp.
- String can be attached to devices to prevent them from falling all of the way to the floor if a patient has a tendency to drop items.
- Soap with a string attached assists the patient who has decreased grasp.
- An electric razor is easier to use, and it also increases the patient's safety. If a patient is on medication that thins the blood, a regular razor should not be used.
- Spray deodorant is easier for a patient with hemiplegia to apply to the noninvolved arm while using the noninvolved hand/arm.
- A brush that attaches to the side of the sink with suction cups can be used for cleaning dentures or to assist a patient who has hemiplegia with washing the noninvolved hand.
- A long-handled skin inspection mirror will be necessary for a patient who has paraplegia or quadriplegia to help the patient prevent pressure sores.

Feeding
- Built-up handles can increase the patient's ability to hold utensils.
- Utensils that are curved or bent can be purchased to enable the patient to bring the utensil to the mouth if the patient demonstrates impaired ROM.
- Swivel spoons can help the patient keep the spoon tipped appropriately to keep food on it if the patient has limitations with supination or motor planning.
- Weighted utensils may help decrease slight to moderate tremors enough to allow the patient to feed him- or her-

self; otherwise, a weight can be placed on the patient's arm to slow tremors but the weight should not be heavy enough to cause fatigue early during the meal.

- Universal cuffs allow a patient with weak grasp to hold utensils.
- A mobile arm support or deltoid aid can be positioned to assist the patient with feeding if the patient has impaired ROM and/or weakness. The patient needs to actively extend the shoulder to lower the device to the plate, but then these devices mechanically assist with shoulder flexion and help remove the effects of gravity on movement.
- Straws can increase the patient's independence with drinking if the patient is unable to lift or hold a cup.
- Cups with a section cut out will allow the patient to tip the cup and drink all the contents if the patient is unable to extend the neck and tip the head back. The cut-out area allows clearance of the patient's nose while tipping the cup.
- Cups can also have one or two handles if the patient demonstrates weakness, and lids can be placed on some cups to prevent spilling if the patient has tremors or weakness.
- Scoop dishes, divided dishes, or plate guards provide a rim for the patient to scoop food against when attempting to get food on the utensil.
- A nonslip mat or damp dishtowel can be used to prevent a plate from sliding away from the patient during feeding.

Home Management
- Built-up grips can be placed on pens and pencils to make writing easier. Other devices that slip on the patient's finger(s) can assist a patient in holding a pen.
- A writing bird, which holds a writing utensil, may be used. This device slides along the table or writing surface, so the patient is not required to hold the device. This will assist a patient who has tremors or weakness.

Assistive Technology

- Paperweights help stabilize writing paper.
- Electric typewriters and computers can make communication easier.
- Bookholders allow a patient to continue reading if he or she is unable to hold a book.
- A mouth stick or electric page turner can assist in turning pages for a patient who has quadriplegia.
- Extended levers can be applied to doorknobs.
- Specialized holders can be attached to telephone receivers, or a voice-activated phone can be installed.
- Faucets can have extensions mounted to make turning easier.
- When organizing the kitchen cabinets, items that are used most frequently should be placed on the lowest shelves or toward the front of the shelves for easy access. Shelves can also be built to pull out from the cabinet or lazy susans can be installed to make the items in the back more accessible. Cabinet doors may also be removed to allow better mobility and function for a patient in a wheelchair.
- A high stool can be placed in the kitchen to allow a patient who has decreased endurance to sit while washing dishes or preparing a meal.
- A utility cart with wheels can assist a patient in transporting items.
- Reachers can aid a patient in removing light items from high shelves. Specialized reachers are able to lift heavier items such as large cans safely; refer to an assistive device catalog.
- Special nonslip mats can be placed under a cutting board or bowl while the patient works.
- A specialized cutting board with two stainless steel nails through its center can assist in holding a vegetable while chopping.
- Countertops can be adapted to achieve the proper work height.

- Light kitchen utensils may be purchased and built-up handles can be added if a patient demonstrates weakness. On the other hand, heavy utensils may also be used if the patient demonstrates tremors or incoordination.
- Electric appliances can be used when possible to decrease the patient's amount of work.
- Oven mitts that extend farther proximally on the patient's arm provide more safety when removing items from the oven.
- Pots and pans with two handles can be used by a patient who demonstrates weakness.
- A specialized pan holder with suction cups helps stabilize a pan on the stovetop.
- A steamer basket can be placed in a pot with boiling vegetables. This allows the patient to remove the basket to strain the vegetables, which erases the need to carry and tip a hot pan.
- A stove with front controls will assist a patient who is in a wheelchair.
- Special loop scissors remain open and require very little force to close in order to cut.
- Special knives, such as a right-angle knife or rocker knife, can be used to make cutting easier.
- Lightweight and easy-to-open containers should be used for food storage. Groceries, such as milk, may need to be purchased in smaller amounts to allow a patient to lift the items independently. Jar openers can assist a patient with decreased grasp.
- Prepared foods that can be heated in the microwave are simple for a patient to make at meal time.
- Cleaning tools such as mops or brooms with flexible handles can be used to prevent bending.
- An adjustable ironing board can allow the patient to sit while working.

Assistive Technology

- Lightweight vacuums or self-propelled vacuums can allow a patient with decreased strength to continue cleaning. Heavier vacuums assist a patient with tremors or incoordination while cleaning.
- A front-loading washer and dryer permit a patient to retrieve all the clothes from the appliance.

Devices for Work and Leisure activities can be located in many catalogs from assistive technology companies. Many devices can be used for specialized tasks; however, these are applicable to patients on a very individualized basis as jobs and leisure activities vary from one person to another. This guide seeks to provide general knowledge, so a therapist seeking this specialized information should complete research independently.

Associated Reactions.   See Reflexes and reactions.

Astereognosis.   See Cognitive-perceptual deficits.

Asymmetrical Tonic Neck Reflex (ATNR).   See Reflexes and reactions.

Ataxia.   An uncoordinated gait characterized by a wide-based, unsteady gait. The patient's steps may be uneven in length or timing, and the patient may have a tendency to walk toward the side that has the lesion site. The patient may also demonstrate little to no arm swing. This specific type of gait occurs following a cerebellar lesion. Treatment should focus on compensatory techniques to allow the patient to complete necessary functional activities.

Athetosis.   Involuntary movement that occurs in slow, wormlike, twisting movements and is usually arrhythmic. The extremities, face, and neck usually demonstrate this deficit; however, the patient does not display athetosis while sleeping. A lesion in the basal ganglia may result in athetosis. See Cerebral palsy for treatment.

ATNR.   See Reflexes and reactions.

Attention. The ability to focus on a task, person, or object without being distracted by other stimuli. See <u>Cognitive-perceptual deficits</u> for further discussion and treatment.

Attention Span. The cognitive ability to focus on a task over an extended period of time. It is impaired in individuals with Attention-Deficit Hyperactivity Disorder (ADHD) and others with impulsivity. <u>Relaxation therapy</u> can be used to help individuals to self-regulate hyperactive behavior that interferes with attention span.

Attention Deficit Disorder (ADD). A condition in which children with average or above average intelligence develop hyperactivity and/or inattention. This condition affects boys more often than girls. The cause is unknown.

Specific Treatments
- Provide vestibular stimulation to decrease hyperactivity
- Complete activities that require bilateral integration/coordination and motor planning
- Utilize activities that increase trunk control and balance through the treatment of antigravity extension, joint stability and/or cocontraction of muscles, and righting and equilibrium reactions
- If using rotational devices for vestibular input, check that the patient has the eyes closed and the head in 30° flexion
- Inhibit increased muscle tone through the use of slow rocking, joint compression, deep pressure or massage, neutral warmth, and low frequency/low intensity vibration
- Increase tactile stimulation to assist with sensory organization/tactile discrimination which can increase the patient's level of alertness; recommended areas of the body include the face, hands, mouth, and soles of the feet
- Teach the patient new ways to complete tasks
- Improve problem-solving by using questioning techniques

- Educate parents on sensory and vestibular techniques that help the child organize the sensory system and increase attention; this allows the parents to apply these techniques at home for carryover of increased attention from one situation (the clinic) to another (the home)
- Establish a behavior modification program, using rewards instead of punishment
- Assist the patient in establishing a system of reminders to improve memory
- Help organize the environment to reduce distractions

Contraindications/Precautions

- Observe changes in behavior while being cognizant of all the patient's medications; monitor side effects
- Follow restrictions that have been set if the patient is using diet therapy
- Monitor the behavior reward program and discontinue use if it is not effective

Attention-Deficit Hyperactivity Disorder (ADHD). Inattention, hyperactivity, and impulsiveness that interfere with a child's, adolescent's, or adult's ability to learn, work continuously, and engage in leisure activities. The disorder also impacts on interpersonal relationships.

Treatment

- Ritalin, a psychostimulant, which is the trade name for methylphenidate hydrochloride, is frequently prescribed for ADHD
- Cognitive-behavioral therapy
- Sensory integration therapy
- Biofeedback
- Relaxation therapy

Auditory Sensation. Receiving, discriminating, localizing, and interpreting sounds through the ears. Examples of damage to auditory sensation are otosclerosis (chronic progressive deafness of low tones), cerebral deafness (caused by brain lesion), and perceptive deafness (caused by damage to sensory receptors of cochlea).

Autism. A disorder characterized by extreme withdrawal, inability to establish relationships with parents or peers, difficulty in communication with others and using language, an inward turning toward self in fantasy, and highly repetitive actions. Specific behaviors observed are lack of awareness of others, absence of social play, lack of eye contact and marked distress over minor changes in the environment. Treatment includes the use of augmentative communication, sign language, behavior therapy, gross motor coordination, computer games, Sensory integration therapy, Music therapy, and Creative arts. The cause is unknown. This condition occurs in a 4:1 ratio of males to females.

Specific Treatments

- Complete gross motor coordination activities to improve gross motor skills
- Increase joint stability and cocontraction of muscles through the use of vestibular linear input (a swing), proprioception, prone extension during play, or sucking
- Increase motor planning skills
- Reduce stress if the patient engages in self-abusive or self-stimulating behaviors through adaptation of the environment for less distractions
- Utilize vestibular activities to facilitate muscle tone (rapid rocking) or inhibit muscle tone (slow rocking)
- Decrease tactile defensiveness through the application of different textures
- Complete mazes to increase both gross and fine motor spatial relations
- Give simple directions for tasks
- Teach Stress management or Relaxation therapy
- Decrease the use of routines over time by encouraging the person to try new situations/activities
- Encourage socialization through community outings, group therapy, or support groups
- Assist the patient with language and communication through the use of a communication board or other device

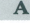

Autism

- Complete <u>Self-care</u> activities to increase self-esteem and independence
- Encourage parallel or cooperative play versus solitary play
- Explore <u>Leisure</u> activities

Contraindications/Precautions

- If using a behavior modification program, understand that the child has difficulty generalizing consequences from one situation to another
- Observe safety precautions when using sensory devices such as the hammock or scooterboard

Autogenic Training. A system of self-regulation of the autonomic nervous system in which the client uses visualization, deep diaphragmatic breathing, and "mind-quieting phrases," such as "my hands are heavy and warm" to reach a relaxed state in treatment of <u>Anxiety</u> and stress disorders. <u>Biofeedback</u> can be combined with autogenic training.

Automatic Stepping. See <u>Reflexes and reactions</u>.

Autonomic Dysreflexia. A sympathetic reflex of the nervous system that can result when uncomfortable conditions or adverse stimuli are introduced to a patient with spinal cord injury; generally those who have a lesion above the level of T_6. The source of the reflex may include any of the following: distended bladder, impacted bowel, pressure sores, ingrown toenails, enemas, catheters, or certain types of muscle facilitation techniques (see <u>Motor control problems</u>). The reflex can result in hypertension, flushing, sweating, pupil constriction, headache, goosebumps, or nasal constriction.

Treatment

- When a patient demonstrates symptoms of dysreflexia, the patient's head should be elevated and the adverse stimuli should be removed. Dysreflexia should be treated immediately as it may result in death.

Aversion Therapy.   A form of behavior therapy in which punishment or unpleasant stimuli, such as creating nausea, are used to extinguish maladaptive behavior such as alcoholism, drug abuse, sexual deviance, and self-mutilation.

Avoidant Personality Disorder.   Characterized by social avoidance, lack of friends, inhibition of feelings, feeling of inadequacy, and hypersensitivity to criticism. Individual tends to be a loner and does not seek out social groups or friendships. Group therapy where the individual has the opportunity to role play and learn social skills is an appropriate treatment approach.

Awareness.   The ability to understand and remember that the self has deficits which limit performance in the affected areas. For example, the patient who has hemiplegia and does not have awareness that his or her left side is paralyzed is at increased risk of falls. The patient may attempt to transfer while unattended since he or she does not recognize that help is required to compensate for the hemiplegia. See Cognitive-perceptual deficits for further discussion and treatment.

Ayurveda.   An ancient Hindu medical practice that strives to improve health by harmonizing mind, body, and spirit. Its name is derived from the Sanskrit meaning life and knowledge. It utilizes prescribed diet, herbal remedies, massage therapy, yoga, and pulse diagnosis. The treatment prescribed is individualized to put the patient in harmony, which helps to prevent illness. Ayurvedic practitioners recommend a daily routine that consists of early rising, prescribed exercises, sensitivity and response to bodily needs such as defecation and sleep, cleaning of body and use of oil massage, and maintaining good mental health and ethical standards.

Babinski's Reflex. See Reflexes and reactions.

Balanced Forearm Orthosis. An assistive device, which is also referred to as a Mobile arm support. See Assistive technology and Mobile arm support for further discussion of adaptive equipment.

Bathing. An activity of daily living (ADL) that is essential to an individual's self-care. See Self-care for specific adaptive techniques, Assistive technology for adaptive equipment, and specific diagnoses/conditions for further discussion and treatment.

Bed Positioning. While in bed, the patient should be positioned to prevent contractures and abnormal tone, maintain skin integrity, decrease pain, and reduce reflexive postures. See Positioning for treatment.

Behavior Rehearsal. Opportunity for clients to practice different social roles to develop the skill of empathy, understanding, or compassion. For example, the client can take the role of a parent, child, or therapist.

Behavior Therapy. The application of treatment techniques based on the principles of learning theories that includes aversion therapy, contingency management, and systematic desensitization. The main purpose is to change maladaptive behavior through positive reinforcement, modeling behavior, and conditioning.

Bibliotherapy. A therapeutic technique in which the therapist recommends books to the patient based on the content of the book and its specific relevance to the patient in working out problems. Reading groups can be incorporated with group therapy.

Bilateral Clasped Activities. A treatment technique by Bobath (1990) to help the patient relearn normal movement with the affected arm by allowing the nonaffected arm to assist the affected arm through movement patterns. The nonaffected arm also provides sensory input and increases the patient's awareness of the affected arm. See Motor control problems, Neurodevelopmental approach.

Bilateral Integration.   The ability to coordinate both sides of the body or both hands or feet while engaging in an activity. It is an important concept in sensory integration therapy. Examples include dancing, skating, hitting a baseball, driving a car with manual transmission, and assembling parts with two tools simultaneously.

Biofeedback.   A treatment method in which the client is taught to become aware of internal processes such as heart rate, blood pressure, finger temperature, or muscle tension as a means to control function. The client learns by using monitoring devices that sound a tone or show a visual display when changes in pulse, blood pressure, brain waves, or muscle contractions occur. Biofeedback is usually combined with Relaxation therapy so that the client can produce beneficial changes in his physiology. The client can apply the information learned from biofeedback to reduce stress. A training program is designed to develop the ability to control the autonomic (involuntary) nervous system. After learning the technique, the client may be able to control heart rate, blood pressure, skin temperature, or to relax certain muscles. Biofeedback has been used successfully in conjunction with Relaxation therapies for clients who experience tension headaches, insomnia, hypertension, Anxiety, chronic pain, Depression, Schizophrenia, and Attention deficit disorders. It has also been used to increase muscle control and for incontinence.

Biopsychosocial Approach.   Implies that an etiology of a disease has biological, psychological, and sociological determinants such as genetic, developmental, and environmental factors. In treatment, biopsychosocial implies a holistic, multimodal treatment approach encompassing occupation, medication, psychological counseling, exercise, nutrition, Stress management, and cultural considerations.

Bipolar Disorder. An affective illness characterized by episodes of mania and Depression. Symptoms of the disorder fluctuate from extreme euphoria, delusions of grandeur, and frantic activity to profound sadness, guilt, lowered self-esteem, fatigue, and suicidal ideation. Cognitive-behavioral approaches have been successful in treating individuals with bipolar disorders. These approaches include Relaxation therapy, Biofeedback, Stress management, and Cognitive therapy.

Blindness. Loss of vision which, when corrected, is no better than 20/200 feet. This term may also refer to a visual field deficit, which results in only 20° of vision from the center of peripheral vision. Persons who are born blind are diagnosed with congenital blindness, while persons who are blind resulting from a trauma or sudden onset of a disease are referred to as newly blind. Causes include diabetic retinopathy, Multiple Sclerosis, conjunctivitis, a detached retina, glaucoma, or pressure on the optic nerve.

Specific Treatments
- Complete gross and fine motor coordination activities to maintain the patient's ROM and use of the hands
- Provide mobility training in the home or work environment
- Teach compensation techniques through the use of the other senses such as hearing or smell
- Educate the patient on devices that can assist with learning such as books on tape or a computer that is voice-activated and talks back to the user
- Address emotional adjustment to the condition
- Increase the patient's self-esteem by completing activities that allow the patient to be successful
- Help the patient reorganize the home to make functional activities easier; for example, reorganize the kitchen to place all necessary items within easy reach
- Increase socialization through community outings or support groups

- Teach the patient skills that will be required for return to work if applicable
- Help the patient develop new leisure interests
- Instruct the patient regarding assistive devices that can help in the home such as talking clocks, timers, etc.

Contraindications/Precautions
- Monitor the patient's safety judgment
- Inspect the home for hazards or dangerous situations
- Educate the patient on other impairments resulting from diabetes, such as decreased sensation and poor circulation, if blindness has occurred as a result of diabetic retinopathy

Body Image.   An individual's subjective concept of his or her physical appearance based on conscious or unconscious feelings toward self.

Body Mechanics.   To prevent future back or other injuries, the occupational therapist should educate the patient on biomechanical principles. These principles assist a patient in positioning him- or herself in postures that reduce the stress placed on the spine or other joints. Proper body mechanics may not only decrease pain or vulnerability to injury, but they also help the patient conserve energy, because it requires more energy to hold an unnatural position. Positions to be avoided include prolonged static flexion or repetitive flexion of the lumbar spine and lifting or carrying objects without maintaining the lumbar curve of the spine. Once the patient understands the underlying principles, the therapist should observe the patient while he or she completes various activities such as <u>Self-care</u>, therapeutic exercise, work simulation, or transfers. The therapist should provide the patient with verbal cues and reminders to incorporate proper body mechanics into regular routines. As treatment progresses, the patient should become more accustomed to the new positions, and he or she should be able to recognize and self-correct poor positions/patterns.

Principles

- Tilt the pelvis slightly anteriorly from neutral when sitting or standing for long periods of time to decrease low back muscle tension.
- When lifting objects, position oneself close to and facing the object to prevent reaching with the upper extremities or twisting of the trunk.
- If a person needs to turn the body, turn with both lower extremities while keeping the trunk in line with the lower extremities. This helps prevent injury from twisting the trunk separately from the lower extremities.
- Use the hip flexor and extensor muscles to lower and raise the pelvis to pick items up from low surfaces, while keeping the back straight. Do not bend at the spine to reach down to the floor.
- Incorporate rest or walking breaks into the routine each hour if the patient has low back pain and is required to sustain static positions for extended periods of time.
- A patient can place one foot on a short stool when standing at the bathroom sink, kitchen counter, etc. This tilts the pelvis slightly posteriorly to relieve pressure since prolonged standing can promote an overemphasized anterior pelvic tilt.
- When sitting, the patient should flex the hips and knees without flexing the spine.
- If the patient is lifting a heavy object, the object should be brought close to the patient's center of gravity. The patient should also balance the weight of the object between both upper extremities. For example, the patient should not carry a heavy book bag over only one shoulder.
- Work surfaces should be adjusted to the proper height to promote good posture and body mechanics. A patient should have the ankles, knees, hips, and elbows near 90° flexion. The wrists and the neck should be in the neutral position.

Body on Body Righting. See Reflexes and reactions.

Body on Head Righting. See Reflexes and reactions.

Body Part Identification. The ability to identify the position of body parts on self or on other persons. See Cognitive-perceptual deficits for further discussion and treatment.

Body Scheme. The perceptual process of being aware of one's body and its integral parts. An individual with hemiplegia can experience difficulty with incorporating the affected site in activities of daily living and can develop neglect. It is assessed by the ability to identify the position of body parts in relation to one another and to objects in the environment. See Cognitive-perceptual deficits for further discussion and treatment.

Borderline Personality Disorder. Marked by an inability to discover meaning in one's life, a feeling of emptiness, and difficulty in maintaining long-term relationships. Emotional outbursts, sadness, fear, and suicidal ideation are frequently experienced. This disorder can lead to substance abuse, domestic violence, criminal behavior and homelessness. Treatment includes medication, Cognitive-behavioral therapy, and Psychoeducational approaches.

Boutonniere Deformity. A digit that demonstrates flexion of the proximal interphalangeal (PIP) joint with hyperextension of the distal interphalangeal (DIP) joint. This condition can result from stretching of the extensor central slip and shortening of the oblique retinacular ligaments.

Bradykinesia. Difficulty carrying out voluntary movement within the usual/normal time span. A patient with this deficit may demonstrate slow eye movements, decreased arm swing during ambulation, or decreased equilibrium or protective responses. A lesion in the basal ganglia may result in bradykinesia. Patients who have Parkinson's disease often demonstrate these symptoms. See Parkinson's disease for treatment and further discussion.

Broca's Aphasia.   See Aphasia.

Brushing.   Using a soft-bristled brush at a very high frequency to help facilitate muscle tone, as hypothesized by
Rood (1964) who used a battery-powered brush. Brushing
should occur for 3 to 5 seconds with 30 seconds between
repetitions. The muscle responds best to the facilitation if
the brushing is completed over the dermatome that is innervated by the same segment which innervates the muscle.
For example, if facilitating the biceps, dermatome C5
should be brushed, as this is the primary segment that
innervates the biceps. The best facilitation occurs while the
brushing is being performed. Areas that have many free
nerve endings should not be brushed, including the face,
head, and ear. Results have shown that the effects last a
very short period of time.
Precautions
- Avoid the use of brushing to the face of patients with
spinal cord injuries or brainstem injuries since it could
result in Autonomic dysreflexia.

See Motor control problems; Rood approach for more discussion of brushing and Facilitation techniques.

Bulimia   is an eating disorder marked by recurrent or continuous episodes of binge eating followed by self-induced
vomiting, fasting, and diarrhea. Individual may engage in
excessive exercise. Many times bulimia is associated with
Anorexia. There are a number of theories to explain the
causes. Generally most researchers and clinicians attribute
bulimia to biopsychosocial factors such as genetics, perfec-
tionist personality patterns, social and societal expectations, family pressures, or hypersensitivity to criticism.
Depression and an overly concern about body shape frequently accompany bulimia. Other symptoms include men-
strual disturbances, tooth decay, and dehydration.

Treatment

- Use of a holistic approach is important in helping the client to realize that psychological, physical, and spiritual issues are related to the onset of symptoms and in the treatment.
- The first step in treatment is to protect the client's health and to remove the symptoms that are life threatening such as starvation and dehydration.
- Hospitalization may be needed to control these factors through special diets and, in some cases, tube feeding.
- Cognitive-behavioral therapy
- Family therapy
- Group therapy

Burn Hand Splint. Resting splint fabricated to prevent a patient from developing a claw hand deformity following a burn to the hand, specifically the dorsal surface. The claw hand deformity results in hyperextension of the metacarpal (MCP) joints, flexion of the proximal interphalangeal (PIP) and distal interphalangeal (DIP) joints, and a flattened palmar arch. The resting hand splint should place the patient's hand in 30° wrist extension, thumb abduction to a functional position, 0° PIP and DIP flexion, and 75° MCP flexion. The prescribed wearing schedule is for the patient to wear the splint at all times unless the patient is bathing or doing hand exercises. See Burns for further discussion and treatment.

Burns. A skin disorder that results in tissue injury. The cause may be from a thermal agent, chemical, or electrical current.

Specific Treatments

- Provide positioning devices to prevent contractures or pain; devices include: foam head donut (prevent neck flexion contracture), foam ear protector (prevent pressure on ear), arm trough (prevent shoulder adduction contracture), and foot board (maintain functional position of ankle)

Burns

- Fabricate splints as needed to prevent deformity and contractures; splints include: soft cervical collar (prevent neck flexion contracture), airplane splint (prevent shoulder adduction contracture), elbow conformer (prevent elbow flexion contracture), wrist cock-up splint (prevent wrist flexion contracture), C-splint (prevent tightening of thumb web space), abductor wedge (prevent hip adduction contracture), knee conformer (prevent knee flexion contracture), and foot-drop splint (maintain functional position of ankle)
- Complete activities that allow the patient to demonstrate success and increase self-esteem
- Avoid the use of chemicals which may irritate the skin
- Assist the patient with finding an alternate way to communicate, such as a communication board, if the patient is intubated
- Complete Self-care activities to maintain functional activity
- Later in therapy, address skills that will be necessary for return to work such as gross and fine motor coordination or muscle strength
- Help the patient develop new leisure interests

Contraindications/Precautions

- Monitor the skin for infection and disinfect splints
- Observe the skin for areas of breakdown or areas where skin grafts have failed
- Monitor ROM for changes that could be due to heterotopic ossification
- Observe for signs of peripheral nerve damage, which may result from compression
- Monitor the scars and treat with scar pads, if needed, to prevent hypertrophic scarring
- Monitor ROM to prevent contractures and provide assistive devices as needed; see recommendations above

Buttonhook.   A piece of adaptive equipment that is useful in assisting a patient in buttoning his or her shirt indepen-

Burns

dently. The patient places the hook through the buttonhole of the shirt, and then the patient positions the hook around the button. While pulling the hook toward the buttonhole, the button is pulled through and the button is fastened. This tool is especially helpful for a patient who has hemiplegia and must fasten buttons with one hand. See Cerebral vascular accident for further discussion and treatment techniques for dressing.

Cancer.   Unregulated cell growth, which may invade surrounding tissue and metastasize to move to other areas of the body. Many types of cancer exist which may occur at any age. The cause is unknown. Unregulated cell growth disrupts the ability of organs to complete their normal functions.

Specific Treatments

- Complete activities to maintain muscle strength, ROM, and endurance
- Fabricate splints and provide positioning devices as needed to prevent contractures and deformity
- Teach Pain management, Stress management, and Relaxation therapy
- Instruct the patient to use energy conservation and work simplification techniques when completing functional activities
- Check the patient's safety judgment and treat as needed
- Encourage the patient to become involved in support groups for socialization and emotional adjustment to the disease
- Take the patient on community outings to elevate mood and increase socialization
- Assist the patient with finding a new means of communication if needed
- Ensure success by grading activities to the patient's ability which will help increase self-esteem
- Address the patient's ability to cope with the disease and problems resulting from its progression
- Complete Self-care activities to maintain functional activity
- Instruct the patient on assistive devices, which can make functional activities easier. devices may be used for dressing, feeding, tub or toilet transfers
- Complete a home evaluation and give recommendations regarding modifications of the environment to increase the patient's safety

Contraindications/Precautions
- Know the patient's medications being used, including radiation and chemotherapy, and possible side effects

Cardiac Dysfunction. A disorder that affects the function of the heart by an adverse condition of the blood, tissue, muscles, or vessels around the heart. Some cardiac dysfunctions include the following: *arteriosclerosis* (also referred to as coronary artery disease), a build-up of plaque on the coronary artery walls which decreases amount of oxygenated blood being delivered to the heart which results in ischemia of heart muscle; *myocardial infarction*, death of heart muscle which may occur from ischemia of heart muscle and cause a decreased ability of the heart to pump blood; *angina pectoris*, chest pain, which often radiates to the left shoulder, jaw, neck, or down the left arm; and *valvular disease*, state of valves becoming fibrous which affects their ability to close completely and results in regurgitation of blood (heart murmur). Patients who receive rehabilitation services are those who are recovering from a myocardial infarction or open heart surgery. Open heart surgery is usually performed to complete coronary artery bypass graft with the goal being to prevent a myocardial infarction by providing more blood to heart tissue if the patient has arteriosclerosis. If the physician chooses to use a less invasive method to decrease arteriosclerosis, balloon angioplasty may be completed. This involves placing a balloon tipped tube into the coronary artery near the point of blockage, and compressing the balloon to help open the artery (Atchison, 1995).

Specific Treatments
- Complete activities to maintain the patient's endurance
- Use resistive activities to maintain muscle strength
- Instruct the patient on energy conservation and work simplification principles
- Educate the patient about stressful situations (see precau-

tions below) which can cause dangerous results, and teach the patient to avoid those situations
- Teach the patient to use good body mechanics
- Train the patient to use <u>Stress management</u> and <u>Relaxation therapy</u> when necessary
- Instruct the patient to use adaptive techniques and/or assistive devices to make functional activities easier
- Set up a schedule for the patient to follow when completing home management activities, which allows for periods of rest between activity
- Complete job simulation if the patient plans to return to work
- Modify current leisure activities or explore new interests

Contraindications/Precautions
- Stressful situations should be avoided
- The patient should use assistive devices rather than bending over to dress or pick up items
- The patient should also use assistive devices or reorganize the home to avoid reaching overhead
- While completing isometric exercise, the patient should be taught to exhale to avoid holding the breath
- Hot, humid environments should be avoided
- The patient should not overexert while exercising
- Cease activity if the following symptoms occur: a cold sweat, glassy stare, dizziness, angina or chest discomfort, fatigue, dyspnea, high systolic or diastolic blood pressure, irregular pulse, palpitations, or pain (especially in the legs)
- Patients who have had open heart surgery should not have resistance against shoulder motion, and they should also avoid horizontally abducting the upper extremities which can pull the incision open.

Carpal Tunnel Syndrome. A condition with the following symptoms: numbness and tingling along the pattern of the median nerve (the thumb, index, long, and lateral half of the ring finger), weakness, and clumsiness. The cause is compression of the median nerve within the carpal tunnel, which occurs from a thickness of the transverse carpal ligament or inflammation of the tendons within the carpal tunnel, most often due to cumulative trauma. Repetitive flexing of the wrist often leads to carpal tunnel syndrome.

Specific Treatments

- Utilize graded activities to gradually increase the patient's hand strength
- Immobilize the wrist with a splint, at 10–20° of extension, to prevent flexion and ulnar deviation
- Practice coordination activities
- Complete tendon-gliding exercises
- Control edema, especially following surgery
- Following surgery, also instruct the patient to complete nerve-gliding exercises
- Provide friction massage to prevent adhesions at the scar site
- Maintain upper extremity ROM through exercise
- Reeducate the affected hand with different textures and sensory stimuli
- Educate the patient on the condition and its cause to help prevent reinjury from repetitive movements
- Teach the patient to use joint protection principles and good body mechanics
- Complete a job site evaluation and make recommendations to prevent reinjury from repetitive trauma
- Adapt tools to prevent tight grasp or bad positioning of the upper extremity
- Explore other occupations and new leisure interests if necessary
- Have the patient wear a splint to help immobilize the wrist at work

Contraindications/Precautions

- Monitor for skin breakdown and pressure areas from the splint

- Instruct the patient that overuse of the affected hand can lead to tenosynovitis

Case Management.   A comprehensive system of treating individuals with mental illness that includes evaluating client needs, developing feasible goals, arranging for services in the community and monitoring client's progress and follow-up. The case manager is concerned with the client's compliance to medication, housing, vocational plan, support group and counseling or psychotherapy.

Catecholamine.   Derived from the amino acid tyrosine, it has a vital function in the brain of stimulating the nervous system, cardiovascular function, metabolic rate, temperature, and smooth muscles. It plays a key role in arousing the autonomic nervous system (sympathetic response). Dopamine and norepinephrine are catecholamines.

Categorization.   The cognitive ability to sort objects into similar or different groups. It entails the ability to generalize and differentiate people, objects, concepts, emotions, and animals. Purposeful activities can be devised by the therapist to stimulate learning, for example, games where the individual sorts pictures into categories or groups.

Catharsis.   A term used by Freud to describe how repressed ideas or traumatic experiences are brought to the consciousness during psychotherapy. In general terms it refers to the free expression of negative feelings, such as fear and anxiety, which are released through expressive media such as art, music, poetry, or Dance.

Central.   See Anatomical Position.

Cerebral Palsy (CP).   A nonprogressive motor disorder resulting from damage to the brain before, during or shortly after birth.
Etiology and Epidemiology. The immediate cause of CP is due to a lesion in the brain usually caused by

anoxia or insufficient oxygen to a part of the brain. There are approximately 500,000 individuals in the United States with this diagnosis. Approximately 1 of every 500 live births will have a diagnosis of CP. Prematurity and low birth weights are both risk factors for CP. With the increasing number of low birth weight infants who live as a result of medical technology the risk for CP has increased. It almost seems ironic that excellent neonatal care is an indirect risk factor for CP. Usually the first sign that brain damage may have occurred is the accumulation of bilirubin in the blood indicated by the presence of jaundice. Other causes of brain damage in the fetus are (a) chemical damage to the fetus from the mother; (b) intrauterine infection during the first trimester of pregnancy; and (c) trauma, poor nutrition, radiation, inadequate pre-natal care, rubella, AIDS, toxoplasmosis (protozoan parasite), or sepsis (toxins in the blood) during the later stages of pregnancy and during labor and delivery.

Diagnostic Types. Traditionally, clinicians categorize CP into four types: Spastic (70% occurrence), Athetoid or dyskinetic (20%), Ataxic (10%) and mixed. Other clinicians categorize CP into two categories Pyramidal or Extrapyramidal. Pyramidal or spastic CP indicates that the lesion was in the motor cortex or cortico-spinal tract. Extrapyramidal or athetoid indicates that the lesion was in the basal ganglia. Ataxic CP usually indicates damage to the cerebellum, which controls posture and balance, running, writing, dressing, eating, playing musical instruments and visual tracking of objects.

Major Areas of Disability and Resulting Handicaps

- **Cognition**: About 1/3 of children with CP are mildly impaired with IQs of within minus 1 standard deviation from the mean. Another third are about minus 2 standard deviations. The remaining third are at the 50th percentile for intelligence or above.

- **Epilepsy or Seizures**: Estimated that between 25 to 50% will have tonic-clonic (grand mal) or partial seizures.
- **Visual Impairments**: Five to 10% of children with CP have visual impairments, such as strabismus (lack of alignment of two eyes), Nystagmus and Hemianopsia.
- **Impaired Hearing**: Frequently occur in children with CP. May cause disability in learning and difficulty in social interactions.
- **Sensory and Perceptual Impairments**: The presence of Astereognosis and abnormal pain sensations may be present.
- **Hydrocephalus**: Occurs in about 7% of children. It is manifested by increased cerebrospinal fluid in the brain.

Treatment

- Motor treatment such as Neurodevelopmental treatment
- Augmentative communication aids such as talking computers and language boards
- Ambulation aids or use of wheelchair
- Activities of daily living aids in eating, dressing, toileting and grooming
- Leisure and play activities to stimulate development and increase socialization skills
- Stress management to help individual to deal with resultant disabilities
- Family therapy and Psychoeducational therapy
- Creative arts therapy to help individual express feelings
- Vocational exploration to help individual to actualize abilities

Cerebral Vascular Accident (CVA).   Decreased blood supply to any part of the brain, which may occur suddenly or gradually. CVAs are often referred to as strokes. The intensity may vary from very small CVAs, which are called transient ischemic attacks (TIAs) and result in very little change of function, to large strokes, which can result in profound and permanent loss of function. Conditions that may cause CVAs include arteriosclerosis, hypertension, heart disease, family history of stroke, or hypercholesterolemia. CVAs result in various symptoms depending on the size and location of the lesion which suffers from decreased blood supply (Ratan, 1997). Symptoms range from decreased sensation and motor ability to decreased memory and cognitive ability. Symptoms often follow a typical distribution depending on the hemisphere that incurred the lesion. Patients who have had CVAs on the left side of the brain usually display right hemiplegia, Apraxia, Aphasia, hemianopsia in the right visual fields, impaired right/left discrimination, memory deficits, and Depression. Patients who have had CVAs on the right side of the brain usually display left hemiplegia, hemianopsia in the left visual fields, left neglect, impulsivity, difficulty with spatial relations and figure/ground, and decreased judgment. A lesion in either hemisphere can result in memory difficulty, decreased attention, and emotional lability. The prognosis for the return of function often depends on when therapy is initiated, the site and extent of the lesion, and the rate of recovery of function. For example, a patient who recovers some function immediately following a stroke has a better prognosis than a patient who experiences no change for some time following the stroke.

Specific Treatments

- Increase independence with ADLs
- Utilize an orientation board or other tools to improve the patient's orientation, and develop aids to assist the patient with memory
- Increase visual tracking and scanning; teach compensation techniques to look to the affected side if the patient demonstrates a hemianopsia or patch one eye to decrease double vision

- Improve tactile sensation and teach safety precautions for sensory loss
- Assist the patient in finding an alternate means to communicate if the patient has aphasia
- Promote proper positioning for safety in swallowing and good body alignment
- Relieve stress to the affected shoulder through the application of a sling, to help prevent subluxation. This treatment is controversial; see Sling for further discussion
- Decrease pain
- Decrease edema through elevation, massage, and ice
- Maintain ROM through PROM of affected upper extremity; make sure the head of the humerus is approximated into the glenoid fossa to increase ROM and decrease pain with movement
- Increase voluntary use of affected upper extremity
- Improve muscle strength, motor planning, and coordination
- Normalize muscle tone on the affected side through facilitation or inhibition techniques
- Increase endurance
- Improve swallowing
- Assist patient with psychological adjustment to condition
- Educate patient on condition/disease process
- Complete a home evaluation and give recommendations for equipment to increase the patient's accessibility and safety in the home
- Explore vocational opportunities as needed
- Assist patient with finding leisure activities
- Complete activities to increase the patient's body symmetry and balance
- Fabricate a splint to prevent contractures/deformity and maintain skin integrity
- Teach the patient to complete inspection of the skin, if the patient is wearing a splint, to prevent skin breakdown

- If the patient demonstrates neglect, instruct the patient to use visual cues and reminders to remember to include the affected side during activities
- Adapt the treatment environment to reduce distractions if the patient has decreased attention
- Complete R/L activities while identifying the side being used to increase a patient's R/L discrimination
- Give simple directions if the patient is unable to follow complex directions
- Work on math problems if the patient will be required to manage the finances independently
- Teach Stress management and Relaxation therapy
- Instruct the patient on assistive devices that may be used to increase the patient's independence with Self-care activities such as feeding, dressing, grooming, tub and toilet transfers
- Have the patient bend the unaffected leg under the affected leg, and use it to assist with swinging the legs off the bed to increase independence with transferring from supine to sit
- Complete a job site evaluation if the patient plans to return to work
- Address homemaking activities such as cooking and cleaning, especially if the patient plans to return home alone
- Work on handwriting if the affected upper extremity is also the dominant hand

Contraindications/Precautions

- Monitor for symptoms of reflex sympathetic dystrophy
- Observe the patient's mood and watch for signs of depression
- Measure ROM and fabricate splints to prevent contractures from abnormal tone
- Do not allow the patient to use abnormal postures and movements; train the patient to attempt normal movement

Chaining. A behavioral therapy technique in which an activity is broken down into task intervals for the client to learn in a sequential manner. *Forward chaining* is carrying the task from the first step until completion. *Backward chaining* starts with the last step in the task and works backward in sequence to the first step. As a treatment technique, the therapist divides a complex skill into smaller, manageable components. The therapist teaches the patient one step of the desired skill at a time. With time, the patient learns all steps of a task, and the therapist slowly removes assistance from each step. The therapist may also chain backward, so that the therapist assists the patient throughout the activity until the final step is reached. The therapist allows the patient to complete the final step until the patient demonstrates success. The therapist will then remove assistance one step earlier, so that the patient completes the final two steps of the activity.

Chiropractic Care. A discipline of health practice that examines the relationship between the structure and position of the spinal column to the onset of diseases, pain syndromes, and neurophysiological effects. Chiropractors emphasize prevention and health maintenance, as well as treatment. The major treatment method is spinal manipulation in which the chiropractor uses his or her hands to mobilize, adjust, manipulate, massage, or stimulate the client's spine. Chiropractic care has been shown to be quite effective in treating individuals with low back pain.

Chorea. Involuntary movement that occurs in quick, jerky, and irregular movements. The face and extremities usually demonstrate this deficit. Lesions of the basal ganglia may result in chorea; however, patients have also displayed this deficit following rheumatic fever.

Chronic Obstructive Pulmonary Disease (COPD). A condition that results in obstruction of the small airways in the lungs; often accompanies asthma, emphysema, or chronic bronchitis. Asthma results in spasms of the airways, which reduce the size of the airways and make breathing difficult. Emphysema is a decreased elasticity in the alveolae and bronchioles, which causes the patient to have difficulty with forced expiration. Chronic bronchitis is inflammation of the bronchii, which increases mucous secretions. Causes of this condition can include smoking, allergies, infections, obesity, or nervous system diseases that weaken muscles of respiration.

Specific Treatments

- Increase the patient's endurance through gradual resistive exercises
- Complete exercises to maintain ROM
- Teach the patient to use pursed lip breathing to slow dyspnea; this technique consists of inhaling through the nose with the mouth closed and exhaling through the mouth with the lips formed in a small circle as if the patient were going to attempt to whistle
- Instruct the patient on principles of energy conservation and work simplification
- Prevent the patient from holding the breath when using force such as while pushing or pulling against resistance; holding the breath will increase the patient's shortness of breath
- Educate the patient on good body mechanics to help the patient conserve energy during activities, since poor posture requires more energy than good upright posture
- Instruct the patient on the possibility of decreased respiration due to chemicals or other hazardous material
- Teach the patient Stress management and Relaxation therapy
- Encourage the patient to join a support group for socialization
- Provide the patient with education regarding assistive devices, which may make functional activities easier
- Complete a home evaluation and make recommenda-

tions for equipment to increase the patient's safety and mobility in the home
- Complete a job site evaluation and make recommendations as needed

Contraindications/Precautions
- Avoid the use of hazardous chemicals and irritants that can cause difficulty with breathing
- Monitor for dyspnea and do not overfatigue the patient while completing endurance training

Circadian Rhythm.   The awake, sleep, and activity cycle in animals during a 24-hour period. Individuals can track their circadian rhythm by recording the average hours of sleep needed during a 24-hour period and their activity level during the day.

Circumduction.   See Anatomical position.

Claw Hand.   A condition in which the MCP joints hyperextend and the PIP and DIP joints flex. This may result from an ulnar nerve palsy, which paralyzes the interossei and intrinsic muscles, or from a burn to the hand. See Hand injuries and Burns for further discussion and treatment.

Client-Centered Therapy.   A type of psychotherapy developed by Rogers (1951), which emphasizes the relationship between the client and the therapist, and empowers the client to facilitate psychological growth. Also known as nondirective therapy.

Clinical Observation.   A method of observing and evaluating the client's verbal and nonverbal behavior in a treatment setting.

Clonus.   Alternating contraction and relaxation of a muscle that results in a twitching movement.

Closed Reduction.   The act of correcting a fracture without surgical intervention. The physician manipulates the fragments back into alignment without having to open the skin. The doctor then immobilizes the fracture with a cast or external fixator until healing occurs. An external fixator is hardware, such as rod, which is applied externally to pins which have been screwed into bone.

Cocontraction. This occurs when both the agonist and the antagonist muscles contract at the same time to achieve stability. Examples would include the cocontraction of the muscles of the neck so that a person's head is held upright or the cocontraction of the muscles in a person's trunk and lower extremities while the person is in Quadruped.

Codependency. An individual's addiction that is shared with a significant other such as a spouse. Addictions such as alcohol, drugs, gambling, or smoking may be reinforced by the codependent individual. Individuals with codependency many times have low self worth, difficulties in relating to others, please others at the expense of self and may have a need to control others. Cognitive-behavioral therapy, Psychotherapy, and Creative arts are effective treatment techniques.

Cognition. The mental activity of perceiving, thinking, reasoning, evaluating, remembering, planning, and making decisions. The act of cognition includes memory (perception, encoding, storage, and retrieval of information), attention, language, and executive functioning. It is assessed by the ability to process information in order to solve problems, draw conclusions, or retrieve data. See Cognitive-perceptual deficits for further discussion and treatment.

Cognitive-Behavioral Therapy. Based on a skills-training approach to treatment where the client learns to self-regulate symptoms. Stress management, Biofeedback, Relaxation therapy, Prescriptive exercise, Progressive relaxation, and Psychoeducational approaches are used by the therapist to help the client to learn techniques to reduce symptoms and to prevent the recurrence of the disease.

Cognitive-Behavioral Therapy (*continued*)

Compliance is an important component in the treatment. The client is an active participant in therapy and the therapist helps the client to monitor improvement.

Cognitive Integration and Cognitive (performance) Components. Term used in the Uniform Terminology for occupational therapist. The abilities to use higher level brain functions in evaluating information. These components include level of arousal, orientation, recognition, attention span, initiation of activity, termination of activity, memory, sequencing, categorization, concept information, spatial operations, problem solving, learning, and generalization.

Cognitive-Perceptual Deficits. A patient may demonstrate difficulty with activities of daily living even though the sensory and motor systems of the patient are functioning normally. In this case, the therapist should focus on cognition and perception, which can also greatly affect an individual's ability to complete activities independently. A patient who has difficulty with storing or processing information may be unable to remember the steps of bathing. Likewise, a patient who cannot integrate sensory input with previous knowledge, which gives meaning to the input, may not be able to understand how to put on a shirt. Deficits may be displayed in the following cognitive areas: Attention, Orientation, Memory, Problem solving, and Awareness. The perceptual areas which may demonstrate deficits include the following: Visual foundation skills (Visual acuity, Visual fields, and Oculomotor function), Body scheme, Right/left discrimination, Body part identification, Finger agnosia, Anosognosia, Unilateral neglect, Position in space, Spatial relations, Topographical orientation, Figure/ground perception, and Apraxia (Limb apraxia, Constructional apraxia, and Dressing apraxia).

Approaches

- The *sensory-integrative approach* uses sensory input to help elicit the desired motor responses; however, this treatment requires a lot of time.

- The *neurodevelopmental approach* (Bobath) helps develop perceptual abilities during its handling and retraining techniques. Many of the techniques, which are specific to this motor control theory, provide sensory input which can be utilized for perceptual functions. During bilateral clasped activities, the patient may be increasing awareness of a neglected limb, body scheme, or position in space. While weightbearing, the patient may be retraining proprioception as well as facilitating muscle contraction.

- The *transfer of training approach* believes that the practice of a particular perceptual task can be generalized to other tasks that require the same perceptual function. If a person practices pegboard designs to increase spatial relations, then those spatial abilities may carry over to a transfer activity (the patient may be able to judge the location of the target chair with better accuracy).

- The *functional approach* is the most common method of rehabilitation of perceptual skills. This approach is based on the principle that repetition and practice of perceptual functions will increase the patient's independence. Rather than practicing specific skills, the therapist educates the patient on his or her deficits and assists the patient in compensating for those losses. The therapist may help the patient establish a routine during dressing which will allow the patient to compensate for Unilateral neglect. As the patient learns the routine, he or she becomes more independent with dressing. The therapist may also adapt the environment or objects being used by the patient in order to increase independence. The room may be arranged to decrease distractions or cues may be written and displayed.

General Treatment Considerations

- All treatment techniques should be practiced since repetition can help increase learning.

- Treatment may begin with a specific activity or in a specific environment; however, when possible, treatment should be generalized and applied during functional activities. Doing puzzles does not help the patient to increase body part identification if that ability is never applied during dressing to help the patient understand the orientation of clothing.

- During cognitive treatment, focus is placed on the *process* the patient uses rather than the specific task.
- Treatment should begin at the patient's level of ability and then increase in difficulty as the patient improves, so the patient is always challenged.

Treatment of Specific Deficits

Attention. The ability to focus on a task, person, or object without being distracted by other stimuli.

- Therapy should occur in an environment with few distractions. As the patient improves, the environment can be gradually "normalized," until treatment is possible in the usual location, such as the main room of the outpatient clinic.
- Treatment may be simple and brief in the beginning, but the therapist may increase the complexity of the treatment activity as well as the duration of treatment as the patient improves.
- Computer activities, which send immediate feedback, may be an effective way to increase the patient's ability to sit and work on a task.
- The therapist can read a random list of letters and ask the patient to identify when a specific letter or letters is read.
- A tape the patient enjoys can be played while the patient works on a task to test if the patient becomes distracted.
- The patient can read a list of words that include the words big and little. The patient can be asked to read either the actual word or the size of the word. For example, when reading the list "BIG, LITTLE, big, LITTLE, big, little", the patient can read the words "big, little, big, little, big, little" or the size "big, big, little, big, little, little".

- The therapist may also ask the patient to complete activities which divide attention. For example, the patient is asked to sort a deck of cards according to color and face cards.

Orientation. The ability to identify information about oneself, including name, place, date, and situation.

- Staff members and family should orient the patient to time, place, person, and situation whenever possible.
- Visual aids can be used such as calendars or individualized orientation boards that list the date, place, person's name, and situation (if desired).

Memory. The ability to store information for immediate recall or retrieval at a later date.

- Compensatory techniques are often used with patients who demonstrate memory deficits. The patient may use signs placed around the patient's room or house to give reminders for activities such as turning off the curling iron, lights, or stove. A notebook may be used to take notes when the patient learns a new task or receives new information. An alarm can be set to remind the patient to take medication. The patient's environment can be labeled to help the patient locate items. For example, kitchen cupboards can be labeled if the patient cannot find items when cooking, or a sign can be placed near the bathroom door if room location is difficult.
- The patient can verbally rehearse information to help increase recall.
- Visual images can be used to help the patient recall information.
- If the patient needs to recall a larger amount of information, he or she can make up a story that ties the information together.
- Mnemonics is the use of letters contained in each word in a list that are then joined together as a word to help abbreviate a large amount of information. For

Cognitive-Perceptual Deficits

example, when using a fire extinguisher, the mnemonic PASS helps a person recall the following steps of use: Pull the pin, Aim at the base of the fire, Squeeze the trigger, and Sweep across the fire in short alternating strokes.

- The therapist may assist the patient in developing motor routines to help the patient retrieve information. For example, the patient always undresses in the same pattern and places jewelry in the same location.
- The PQRSTA method includes the following tasks: *preview* material, *question* what will be included, *read* the material, *state* what was read, and *test* by *answering* questions about the material.

Problem Solving. The ability to apply current knowledge in order to create solutions when new problems or situations arise.

- The therapist should provide the patient with various problems and puzzles to solve. Practice will help the patient find helpful strategies.
- <u>Chaining</u> may be used to break a complex problem into smaller, manageable components. If the patient is attempting to balance a checkbook, the therapist can have the patient complete one entry at a time and then check the patient's work to catch errors while the patient still has the problem in mind.
- Group treatment for problem solving may help the patient find new strategies as well as help the patient generalize strategies to new situations.
- The patient can be taught the process for problem-solving as follows:
  - Define the problem
  - Develop possible solutions
  - Choose the best solution
  - Execute the solution
  - Evaluate the outcome

Awareness. The ability to understand and remember

that one's self has deficits which limit performance in the affected areas.

- Feedback from the therapist, or peers if group therapy is used, is an effective means of helping the patient gain awareness regarding behavior.
- The therapist may use role reversal to help the patient see how behavior is viewed by others.
- Self-evaluation encourages the patient to view his or her actions and behavior.

Visual Foundation Skills. These skills are comprised of visual acuity, visual fields, and oculomotor function. *Visual acuity* is the ability to focus on objects both at near and far distances. A person with intact *visual fields* must be able to see objects in each of the four quadrants of vision with each eye. *Oculomotor function* is movement of the eye ball which is caused by the muscles attached to the eye. The four parts of oculo-motor function include range of motion, pursuits, convergence, and alignment.

- A patient with decreased Visual acuity may first bene-fit from a pair of corrective lenses.
- The therapist can help adapt the environment to increase a patient's ability to see. The patient can identify the objects used in the environment that cre-ate the most difficulty, then the therapist make adap-tations to increase the background contrast. For exam-ple, if a patient is unable to see the edge of steps, the therapist can outline the edge of the step with brightly colored tape or paint.
- An increase in illumination may increase the patient's ability to see objects; however, the therapist should attempt to avoid an increase in glare or shadows. Recessed lighting increases shadows and should not be used. The best source of illumination is fluorescent lighting and halogen lamps. When reading, the recom-mended lamp is the 50-watt halogen desk lamp.

Cognitive-Perceptual Deficits

- Patterned backgrounds decrease acuity; highly patterned objects such as rugs, bedspreads, placemats, countertops, and furniture should be modified or replaced with solid colored items.

- A patient with a <u>Visual field</u> cut should be trained to turn the head to the affected side in order to see the missing field. Rehabilitation should focus on the patient's speed when scanning to the affected side, as well as the patient's ability to scan the entire scope of the affected area. This type of compensation is particularly important if the patient wants to resume driving.

- The therapist can provide the patient with specific techniques to help with reading. A green line drawn on the left margin (GO) and a red line on the right margin (STOP) can help the patient identify where the text of a line starts or stops. A patient who has difficulty staying on line while reading can place a ruler or straight edge below the line.

- If a patient has problems keeping text on line while writing, the patient should be taught to focus on the pen tip constantly to ensure the writing does not cross a line.

- Activities that require scanning can help increase the patient's visual attention. Treatment for attention and scanning is most effective when the patient is required to touch or name the object. Objects can be enlarged on a screen to facilitate scanning and head turning.

- Matching activities help increase visual attention as the patient must identify similar or contrasting details.

- The patient can practice the above skills, but the patient should then practice applying those skills in more functional circumstances. The patient can practice scanning when getting clothes out of the closet. <u>Visual acuity</u> may be practiced in the community, for example, while crossing a busy street or searching for items in a grocery store. The patient may attempt to read the newspaper or look up telephone numbers using compensatory techniques for a visual field cut.

Body Scheme. The ability to identify the position of body parts in relation to one another and to objects in the environment.

- Puzzles of the human body may help the patient learn the arrangement of body parts in relation to one another.
- Sensory stimulation to the affected extremities helps the patient increase awareness of the affected side.

Right/Left Discrimination. The ability to differentiate between the right and left sides of the body

- The patient who is not able to spontaneously identify right and left will need to learn compensatory techniques, such as using the wedding ring to help identify the left side of the body.
- Activities that stress the differentiation of right from left may help train the patient in this skill. The patient can be asked to identify body parts on the left or right side of his body. The patient can also be asked to find objects located on the right or left side of a page or activity.
- Sensory input can be increased to the right or left side of the body while asking the patient to identify the side.

Body Part Identification. The ability to identify the position of body parts on oneself or on other persons.

- The therapist can touch one of the patient's body parts and then ask the patient to verbally identify which part was touched.
- The therapist can then name a specific part of the body and ask the patient to touch the desired part.

Finger Agnosia. The inability to name or identify a specific finger when asked to discriminate between fingers, usually during a sensory evaluation.

- Rubbing the patient's affected dorsal surface of the forearm and hand as well as both the dorsal and ventral surfaces of the fingers (usually completed for a minimum of 2 minutes) helps increase the patient's awareness of the fingers.

- Deep pressure (again completed for usually a minimum of 2 minutes) can be applied by placing a hard, rough cone in the patient's hand. This pressure sensation may help the patient identify his or her fingers.

Anosognosia. The inability to perceive that hemiplegia is present following a lesion.

- If a patient consciously denies that hemiplegia has resulted from a stroke, treatment will not be successful.
- As the patient recovers, increased sensory stimulation, verbal cueing, and activities that focus on the affected side (such as self-ROM) may help increase the patient's awareness of hemiplegia.

Unilateral Neglect. The inability to sense or perceive stimuli that are presented on the side of the patient's body which is contralateral to the site of the brain lesion. For example, the patient who has had a right CVA may not dress his or her hemiplegic left arm or turn toward the left to look for food on the left side of the plate.

- Treatment may begin with the practice of visual scanning tasks. The patient can complete cancellation tasks, which require the patient to cross out a particular letter or symbol in a list of random letters/symbols. The activity could then proceed to crossing out a particular word in a paragraph. The task can be graded so that the final step requires the patient to cross out a particular letter in a paragraph.
- Activities that focus on the affected extremity may help increase awareness. Weightbearing, handling, verbal cueing, and repetitive tasks may help call attention to the neglected side.
- The therapist and other staff should approach the patient from the affected side to help the patient learn

to turn toward that side. Also, the patient's room can be rearranged to force the patient to turn toward the affected side to watch television or to see who is entering the room.

- Occasionally, a patient who has left neglect may have a patch placed over his or her right eye to further encourage the patient to look to the affected side.

- If using an adaptive approach, items should be placed on the unaffected side and the therapist should also position on that side so the patient is able to see everything easily during treatment.

- The therapist may need to draw a green line on the left side of the page or a red line at the right margin of the page to help cue the patient when or where to return to the next line while reading. Without these cues, the patient most likely will miss part of the text and be unable to understand the material being read.

Position in Space. The ability to understand terms which define position (e.g., over, under, above, beneath, beside, in front of, in back of) and then apply those positions to objects.

- The patient may complete activities that require spatial abilities such as pegboard designs, block designs, or puzzles. Then the patient can answer questions about objects, such as which block is under, over, above, below, beside, and so on.

- Functional activities that can help increase the patient's sense of position include organizing a closet or cupboard while following the therapist directions to place certain items in certain places.

Spatial Relations. The ability to determine the position of objects in relation to each other or to oneself.

- Walking along a path may help the patient orient him- or herself to other objects.

- The therapist can ask the patient questions about the patient's self in relation to other objects in the room.

Topographical Orientation. The ability to move from one location to another without assistance.

- The therapist can place markers or cues along a path to help the patient learn routes from one place to another. For example, a patient who is in a rehabilitation unit can use different colored signs to find his or her way to occupational, speech, or physical therapy. The therapist may also draw a simple map of the hospital floor or wing, which the patient can follow between therapy clinics. In a long-term care setting, the therapist may place a colored piece of tape on the floor from the dining room to the patient's room to help the patient find the way back from meals independently.
- Once the patient increases these skills, the therapist may attempt the use of verbal maps or instructions to help guide the patient to new locations.
- The patient especially benefit from the memorization of routes that are used the most often.
- If the patient's difficulty with topographical orientation stems from visual deficits or neglect, then treatment should begin with those deficits.

Figure/Ground Perception. The ability to discriminate between an object and its background.

- Treatment may begin by having the patient locate objects in pictures taken from magazines and books. This activity should be graded according to the patient's ability to prevent the patient from becoming frustrated. As the patient improves, the activity can be made increasingly difficult. (The Waldo books are excellent final activities for figure/ground perception.)
- Scanning activities such as word search puzzles can help the patient learn to identify words within a complex background.
- The therapist may need to adapt the patient's environment so that background is simple and objects that are difficult for the patient to see are brightly marked.

Apraxia. A perceptual deficit that hinders patients from completing functional or purposeful movement even though the patient demonstrates normal sensory, motor, and coordination skills

- A patient with ideomotor or ideational apraxia will benefit from the therapist manually guiding the patient's limbs while completing an activity. This method is often referred to as "hand-over-hand."
- Increased tactile and proprioceptive stimulation may facilitate the proper motor movements.
- Chaining is the act of dividing complex activities into smaller, manageable components. The patient can learn each small step of an activity separately, and then combine the small steps into a larger activity once the patient has demonstrated competence with each small step.
- Visualization of the desired motion or activity may assist the patient with motor planning.
- Verbal instruction may be used minimally, but the patient may not understand due to aphasia.
- Treatment should occur in the environment where the desired activity is usually completed. For example, the steps of cooking should be practiced in a kitchen area rather than at a table in an outpatient clinic.
- Patients who have demonstrated constructional apraxia may benefit from visual cues when constructing or drawing designs.
- The therapist can have the patient copy block or peg-board designs, and the therapist should increase the difficulty of the designs as the patient improves.
- Functional activities should be used whenever possible because learning may be task specific in some cases, particularly with individuals who have brain injury. A patient with constructional Apraxia can practice making a sandwich or folding laundry and putting it back into the dresser and closet.

Cognitive-Perceptual Deficits

- Patients who have dressing <u>Apraxia</u> benefit from learning a specific pattern of dressing. The therapist can then teach the patient to use visual cues such as the zipper of pants or the label in a shirt to help orient clothing. Through repetition, the patient will learn dressing. The patient should then use different clothes while using the same visual cues to help orient the clothing so that the technique can be generalized to all pants and/or all shirts.
- Individuals may have difficulty performing activities of daily living such as dressing, grooming or bathing.
- Use the remedial or transfer of training approach where the therapist works with the patient on using compensatory movements.
- Neurodevelopmental methods are also used by therapists in improving dressing skills. In general therapists use functional and adaptive approaches to help the patient to be as independent as possible in performing self-care activities.

Astereognosis. The inability to identify objects through touch or tactile sensation.

- Treatment should begin while allowing the patient to touch and feel an object while looking at it. The next step is blocking the patient's vision while the patient continues to feel the object, so the patient cannot use visual cues for identification. The final step involves placing a pad or towel on the table while the patient continues to feel the object, so the patient is not able to use auditory cues for identification.
- As the patient demonstrates progress, the patient should be asked to identify features of the objects without visual cues. Objects that have opposite or very dissimilar traits should be presented to the patient. For example, the patient can learn to discriminate between a rough and smooth texture.
- The next step involves the identification of a esti-

mated number of objects. For example, the patient is asked to place his or her hand in a bowl and estimate how many marshmallows are in the container.

- The patient can learn to discriminate between large and small objects hidden in a container of sand. Another discrimination task may require the patient to differentiate between two-dimensional and three-dimensional objects.
- The final step of treatment occurs when the patient selects a small object from a collection of several objects and is able to identify the object with vision blocked.
- Treatment may also progress in the following manner:
  - visual examination of the object
  - tactile examination with the unaffected hand while observing
  - tactile examination with both hands while observing
  - tactile examination with the affected hand while observing
  - tactile examination with the unaffected hand with vision blocked
  - tactile examination with both hands with vision blocked
  - tactile examination with the affected hand with vision blocked.
- After the patient is able to successfully identify various objects using this method, two objects can be hidden in a tub of rice or sand. The patient is then asked to retrieve a particular object from the tub.

Cognitive Therapy. First conceptualized by Beck (1976), is defined as a verbal therapy that helps the client to examine his or her thoughts, impulses, and feelings that are contributing to a disorder. The first principle of cognitive therapy is that the way people structure a situation determines how

Cognitive Therapy *(continued)*

they feel and behave. For example, if a person interprets a situation as dangerous, he or she feels anxious and prepares to protect him- or herself. Behavioral techniques are used by cognitive therapists to help clients develop new approaches in dealing with everyday activities by helping them to monitor their behavior and to try out new behaviors.

Cogwheel Rigidity.   A type of rigidity characterized by a rhythmic relaxation and contraction of muscles during passive movement. When moving a body part that has cogwheel rigidity, the part may be difficult to move at first, but then both agonist and antagonist muscles will relax so that movement is easier. However, the muscle Cocontraction will again occur, making movement difficult. This contracting and relaxing will occur many times while the therapist moves the part through its ROM, so that movement feels like it keeps "catching." See Rigidity and Lead pipe rigidity for further discussion.

Color Agnosia.   The inability to name or identify a color. See Cognitive-perceptual deficits for treatment of similar perception disorders.

Community Mental Health Center (CMHC).   An outgrowth of the Community Mental Health Center Act of 1963. The CMHC was conceptualized as an alternative to long-term institutionalization for individuals with mental illness. CMHCs provide five basic mental health services: inpatient hospitalization when needed, outpatient care, partial hospitalization, emergency mental health services, and consultation and education to community groups and agencies.

Community Support Program (CSP).   An initiative of the National Institute of Mental Health in response to the deinstitutionalization of individuals with chronic mental illness. CSP supplied funds to public hospitals, community mental health centers, and county and social service agencies to provide comprehensive services including psychosocial rehabilitation to those with chronic mental illness. Community support system (CSS) was a major thrust of CSP.

Community Support System (CSS). A model that tries to meet the needs of individuals with mental illness, such as health and dental, housing, income support, entitlement (Medicare, Medicaid), and employment, through a case management approach.

Complementary Medicine. Another term for alternative medicine. It refers to the innovations in or alternative approaches to traditional medicine. Relaxation therapies, body work, humor, and therapeutic use of vitamins and herbs are examples of complementary medicine.

Compression. A technique used to help reduce and control edema. See Edema for further discussion and treatment method.

Concentric Contraction. See Contraction.

Concept Formation. The cognitive ability to organize a variety of information to form thoughts and ideas such as the concept of an object (e.g., plane), values (e.g., altruism), and religion (e.g., Hinduism). Concept formation is a higher order cognitive ability that entails learning, memory, and generalization. Group activities such as Values clarification can be used to clarify and facilitate concept formation.

Conduct Disorders. A psychosocial disorder that is sometimes classified as a Developmental disability that is characterized by persistent anti-social behaviors including aggression toward others, destruction of property, theft, dishonesty and illegal violation of rules. The behaviors have a significant negative effect on interpersonal relationships, school achievement and ability to work. Oppositional defiant disorder which includes symptoms of angry and resentful behavior, poor self-control, argumentativeness,

Conduct Disorders

Conduct Disorders *(continued)*

defiance, and vindictiveness is related to conduct disorders and can result in sexual acting out, illegal drug use, delinquency, and running away from home.

Treatment

- Sports programs that allows individual to express feelings in a socially accepted activity
- Social skills training that develops empathy and compassion toward others
- Prescriptive exercise that is meaningful to the child or adolescent and can be incorporated into his or her everyday life
- Stress management to help individual to develop relaxation strategies
- Family therapy to engage family in dynamics of treatment
- Nutritional and diet education
- Volunteer work in the community to develop compassion for others and a sense of responsibility
- Upward bound program to challenge individual and create opportunities for cooperating with others in hiking, camping and mountain climbing
- Creative arts therapy to help individual express feelings in a non-judgmental environment

Constructional Apraxia.   See Apraxia.

Contingency Management.   A group of techniques used in behavior therapy in which the client establishes a contract with the therapist to modify a behavioral response by shaping the consequences of that response. For example, the client will receive a token for positive interpersonal communications.

Continuous Quality Improvement (CQI).   A systems approach to improving the quality of care of an organization, hospital, or agency. In this approach, creativity, trial and error, individual leadership, and achievable and measurable goals are emphasized.

Contraction.   An increase in the tone of a muscle, which may or may not result in the shortening or lengthening of the muscle.

Types of Contractions
- **Isotonic Contractions**: A contraction that results in movement of a body part. Isotonic contractions can be further classified as:
  - *Concentric Contractions*: A muscle contraction that results in shortening of the muscle fibers which are contracting and motion in the direction of the muscle's pull. For example, when the biceps contract, the fibers pull upward (toward the shoulder), resulting in the shortening of the muscle, which causes the forearm to be pulled toward the shoulder (elbow flexion).
  - *Eccentric Contractions*: A muscle contraction that results in elongation of the muscle fibers which are contracting and motion in the opposite direction from the muscle's direction of pull (from what is normally expected during a contraction). For example, when the biceps contracts, the expectation would be a shortening of the muscle, which would cause elbow flexion. However, if the elbow is already flexed against gravity (such as when the patient is sitting upright), the biceps performs an eccentric contraction to return the elbow to full extension. The triceps does not need to actively complete extension, since gravity would normally pull the arm into extension if the biceps was not contracting. Instead, the biceps continues contracting while slowly lengthening to slowly lower the elbow into extension.
- **Isometric Contractions**: A contraction that does not result in movement, but is usually completed for the stabilization of a body part or object.

Contracture.   A shortening of soft tissue or connective tissue that limits ROM at a joint. Positioning and PROM should be used to help prevent contractures; however, contractures may be unavoidable in some instances due to some disease processes. In that case, positioning should be used so that the contractures occur in a functional position, so that the patient is still able to complete functional activities in the presence of limited ROM. The functional position of the hand is slight wrist extension (10° to 30°) with the thumb abducted and slightly flexed and the fingers flexed through partial ROM. This allows the patient to place and hold items in the affected hand or use the hand to assist in activities such as dressing. If the hand contracts while fully flexed, the patient will develop sores in the palm from the fingernails and cleansing the hand will be very difficult. If the hand contracts while fully extended, the patient will not be able to use it to assist with holding or stabilizing objects.

Contraindication.   A condition or previous diagnosis that makes a specific type of treatment dangerous or counterproductive. For example, a patient who has hemiplegia may benefit from neuromuscular electrical stimulation (NMES) to help reeducate the affected muscles. However, if the patient has a pacemaker, the electrical current can cause failure of the pacemaker to respond to cardiac problems. In the case of a patient who has both hemiplegia and a pacemaker, NMES should not be used. Contraindications for treatment are listed following treatment techniques throughout the text.

Contrast Bath.   A type of hydrotherapy that is used to help decrease edema and hypersensitivity through immersion of the affected extremity into alternating warm and cold baths. See Edema for specifics of treatment and further discussion.

Controlled Breathing. Learning to use abdominal muscles in breathing slowly with the aim of reducing stress and anxiety.

Coordination

Coordination.   The ability to control muscle contractions to produce smooth movement with appropriate speed, rhythm, muscle tone, postural tone, and accuracy. To produce controlled movement, the patient must have the appropriate muscles contracting to move a body part as well as to stabilize the joint. Also, he or she will have difficulty with coordination if the patient has perceptual deficits with proprioception, position in space, body scheme, or spatial relations. Coordination may be further subdivided into Gross motor and Fine motor coordination. Gross motor coordination is the ability to control the contraction of large muscles and groups of muscle to complete large, less specific movements. Fine motor coordination is the ability to control the contraction of small muscles to complete fine, precise movements. Below is a list of treatment methods to help a patient increase the control of movements.

Treatment Methods

Gross motor

- Sliding or tossing bean bags toward designated targets
- Placing clothespins onto a vertical or horizontal rod
- Light homemaking tasks such as making a bed or setting a table
- Folding laundry
- Stacking cones
- Reaching for items above the head
- Playing catch
- Pulleys—this activity is especially good for teaching the patient bilateral coordination with both upper extremities
- Ring tree—the patient may use one or both extremities to retrieve one ring at a time from a horizontal rod on one side of the "tree" and move it to a horizontal rod on the other side of the "tree"
- Placing and removing items from shelves
- Light cooking activities which involve opening containers, cutting, and stirring
- Balloon volleyball

- Large tabletop board games like giant checkers
- See Range of motion treatment methods

Fine motor

- Flipping cards
- Manipulating coins
- Theraputty with small objects in putty to be removed
- Tying shoes
- Buttoning buttons
- Pegboard activities
- Lacing
- Chaining links
- Cutting
- Writing
- Board games including checkers, dominoes, Operation, Perfection
- Puzzles
- Opening containers
- Make pasta necklaces/bracelets
- Needlework or knitting
- Crafts such as making tile trivets or painting
- Dialing a telephone

Coping Skills. An individual's ability to self-regulate stress and master the environment. Stress management is an example of a coping skill where the individual becomes aware of the stressors that trigger symptoms and the copers that are helpful in reducing the symptoms. Stress management techniques include Relaxation therapy, Biofeedback, and Prescriptive exercise.

Coronal plane. See Anatomical Position.

Course. The predicted stages of an illness based on clinical observations of the illness and epidemiological studies of stages in an illness. For example, 90% of individuals who have a single manic episode experience future episodes.

Coordination

Another example is the progressive nature of Alzheimer's disease where the individual deteriorates in stages.

Creative Arts. The creative arts include the use of art, music, dance, drama, poetry, and crafts as therapeutic and purposeful activities for the client. In designing a creative arts therapy program the therapist should consider the interests of the client, the goals of treatment, the cognitive level, and the feasibility of implementing the treatment. In general, the creative arts should allow the client to express his or her feelings, attitudes and problems in a free uncensored environment. The creative media should enable the client to be spontaneous for example in drawing a dream, in acting out a personal conflict, in expressing emotion through dance or creating a poem expressing a feeling. The therapist tries to guide and encourage the client to use the creative media in a meaningful way. The interpretation of the client's finished product can be done jointly with the client. It can help the client in gaining insight into conflicts and emotional problems by tying together the process of completing the creative expression and the client's attitude toward the product. The creative arts have also been an important area for occupational therapists to embed physical goals such as coordination, muscle strength, range of motion and perceptual motor into a purposeful activity.

Crepitus. A creaking or grating sound and feeling which occurs at a joint during movement; this sensation often accompanies movement at arthritic joints.

Crisis Intervention. A 24-hour service that is made available to clients with mental illness to reduce the stress on the client or family members. Problems such as a loss of job, broken friendships, drug-related problems, or criminal offenses can many times put the individual into a crisis. A case manager or mental health professional can provide support by linking the individual to resources in the

Crisis Intervention *(continued)*
community. Telephone hot lines open and accessible to the individual can be extremely important in alleviating a crisis.

Criterion.   A standard of performance that is the basis or yardstick for comparisons.

Criterion-Referenced Test.   A test based on standards of performance, competence, or mastery, rather than on comparison to a normative group.

Crossed Extension.   See Reflexes and reactions.

Crossing the Midline.   The ability to move arms and legs across the body, coordinated with one's eyes in controlled goal directed actions. Examples include putting on one's socks and shoes, buttoning one's shirts, playing checkers, doing a picture puzzle, playing the piano, and assembling parts.

Cryotherapy.   The application of cold temperature through compressed ice packs or sprays to relive pain, reduce spasticity, and reduce tissue swelling, such as in sprains to muscles or ligaments. See Physical agent modalities for further discussion and treatment.

Culture-Free Test.   A test that is not culturally biased and can be administered across cultures.

Cumulative Trauma Disorders.
• **Carpal Tunnel Syndrome.** A condition with the following symptoms: numbness and tingling along the pattern of the median nerve (the thumb, index, long, and lateral half of the ring finger), weakness, and clumsiness. The cause is compression of the median nerve within the carpal tunnel which occurs from a thickness of the transverse carpal ligament or inflammation of the tendons within the carpal tunnel, most often due to cumulative trauma. Repetitive flexing of the wrist often leads to carpal tunnel syndrome. The patient may be educated on body mechanics and

ergonomics to help decrease the stress on the affected area. See <u>Carpal tunnel syndrome</u> for further discussion and treatment.

- **Cubital Tunnel Syndrome.** This condition results from compression of the ulnar nerve within the cubital tunnel which is formed by the ulnar collateral ligament, the trochlea, the medial epicondylar groove, and the triangular arcuate ligament. The patient may complain of severe pain, decreased grip and pinch strength, or decreased fine motor coordination. Repetitive motion which requires constant grip may result in this condition. Rest, anti-inflammatory medication, and modalities, such as ultrasound, which decrease swelling around the nerve may be applied as conservative treatment or as adjunct treatment following surgery to release the cubital tunnel. The patient should receive ergonomic education to help decrease the stress to the affected area which has occurred from cumulative trauma.

Cylindrical Grasp.   See <u>Grasp</u>.

Dance. Movement using a series of rhythmical motions and steps. It is a good form of exercise and expression of emotions.

Dance Therapy. The use of dance or movement as a carefully guided tool to release tension, develop awareness, acceptance of self and for effective social interactions (Hood, 1959; Levy, 1988).

Day Treatment Centers (DTCs). Previously referred to as day hospitals were established in the United States in the 1950s for individuals who were discharged from mental hospitals and could potentially benefit from a period of transitional services. The services provided are comprehensive and include medication management, counseling, group therapy; and occupational therapy. The occupational therapist plays an important role in the DTCs in helping individuals in the performance areas of Work, Self-care, and Leisure. A guiding philosophy of the DTC is to treat the individual as a member of the community where he or she lives.

Debridement. A treatment method used to remove dead tissue and foreign matter from a healing wound. The therapist may choose to place the patient's affected area in a whirlpool prior to debridement, as the moving water helps to soften and loosen the tissue. The therapist then carefully removes the dead tissue with a tweezers, scissors, or scalpel while being very careful to leave all healing/living tissue intact. Hand therapists are those most likely to work with traumatic injuries that require debridement. See Hand injuries for further discussion and treatment.

Decubitus Ulcer. A sore that develops from the positioning of the patient. Patients who require total or maximal assistance for bed mobility or repositioning in a wheelchair can develop pressure areas on the sacrum or heels of the feet. Prolonged pressure results in decreased circulation to an area, which then causes sores or open areas of the skin. Equipment, such as air mattresses/cushions, water cushions, or gel cushions, to help relieve pressure may be purchased. Bony prominences may also be padded for protection. Special boots or elbow pads may be used while the patient lies in bed. Patients who are specifically at risk are patients who have a spinal cord injury that has resulted in decreased sensation in the lower extremities. If a patient is able to push up from the armrests of the wheelchair or roll from one side to the other, the patient should be instructed to relieve pressure 1 minute for every 30 minutes if possible. Otherwise, nursing staff should set up a schedule to turn the patient while the patient is in bed to help prevent ulcers.

Deep.   See Anatomical position.

Deep Tendon Reflexes.   See Reflexes and reactions.

Deinstitutionalization.   The process of discharging individuals from large state or county hospitals into community facilities such as day treatment centers or supportive housing such as halfway houses, group homes, and residential treatment centers.

Delusion.   A false belief without substance such as believing that people are reading one's mind, or food is being poisoned, or people are plotting against the individual.

Dementia.   A broad term that refers to progressive chronic disorders of the brain characterized by memory loss, confusion, disorientation, personality deterioration, and a complete breakdown in Self-care functions. Alzheimer's disease, Pick's disease, Huntington's chorea, and Organic brain syndrome associated with alcoholism can lead to dementia.

Dependent Personality Disorder.   Describes an individual with an extreme need to be taken care of by another individual. The disorder usually begins in childhood and is characterized by passivity, submissiveness, indecisiveness, poor self-confidence, and a need to be nurtured and supported.

Depression. A mood disorder that can be characterized as mild, moderate, or severe. Symptoms of depression include eating dysfunction, sleeping disturbance, fatigue, low self-esteem, inability to concentrate, difficulty in making decisions, feelings of hopelessness, loss of libido, and sadness. See Dysthymic disorder. Although feelings of depression are universal it is diagnosed as an illness when it interferes with an individual's ability to work or attend school, engage in Leisure activities, attend to Self-care activities, and maintain family and social relationships. Approximately 25% of a given population will experience a clinical depression sometime during their lifetime. Depression is considered to have a biological cause that is linked to the depletion in the body of the neurotransmitter serotonin. Precipitating factors implicated in depression are related to loss such as the death of a close friend or relative, loss of a job, financial loss, divorce or separation, disabling illness or disease, school or work failure, or inability to achieve personal goals. Predisposing factors can include genetic predisposition such as personality traits where the individual is unable to deal with severe environmental or personal loss.

Course of illness. Bouts or episodes of depression can last for weeks, months, or years. A vicious cycle of depression can occur when the depression "feeds upon itself" by dragging the individual into deeper and deeper holes where suicide can be a real threat to the individual. The vicious cycle starts with sleep disturbances that can cause fatigue, and low energy levels leading to an inability to work or attend school causing further withdrawal from social interactions that can lead to a deepening of the illness accompanied by low self-esteem, Anxiety, and suicidal ideation.

Treatment. Each intervention into an episode of depression is critical to prevent the downward spiral that accompanies the course of the illness. A holistic approach is recommended, including medication, exercise, nutrition, Creative arts, individual or group counseling/psychotherapy, vocational counseling, Stress management, Relaxation therapy, Leisure, occupation counseling, and bibliotherapy.

Guidelines for Occupational Therapy. (Stein & Cutler, 1998)

- The cognitive-behavioral approach that emphasizes individuals learning and applying stress management skills, relaxation therapies, exercise, and leisure occupation in their everyday schedules. The therapist works with individual in designing realistic goals and helps the individual to monitor compliance to the therapeutic program.
- Consider cultural values and interests of individual in designing a therapeutic program.
- Use activities and creative media to increase self-esteem, express and channel anger, build lifelong leisure interests, and help individual to gain self-insight.
- Establish a stress management program for individual to identify symptoms that are triggered by stress situations that provoke stress and coping activities that reduce stress.
- Establish exercise program with client considering his or her physical fitness, sports or exercise interests, intensity, and frequency and duration of exercise. Consider feasibility of doing exercise in individual's home, neighborhood, or sports center.
- Consider using Role playing or adopted psychodrama with client in rehearsing stressful or anxiety provoking situations or as part of group therapy sessions.

Depth Perception. The ability to determine the relative distance between one's self and an object. This skill is particularly important in driving a car. See Cognitive-perceptual deficits for further discussion and treatment.

Dermatome. An area of the skin innervated by a specific spinal nerve root. For example, the C4 spinal root provides

Dermatome. *(continued)*
sensation to the area of skin over the shoulders, across the chest from near the clavicle to an imaginary line drawn horizontally between the highest point of the axillae, and a corresponding area over the superior part of the back above the scapulae.

Desensitization. A method of treatment, used with patients who are hypersensitive, to help increase the patient's tolerance of uncomfortable, irritating stimuli. See <u>Sensory deficits</u>, <u>Hypersensitivity</u> for specific treatment methods.

Developmental Disability. A lifetime disability diagnosed before the age of 22, that affects cognition and adaptive behavior. It may include conditions such as <u>Mental retardation</u>, <u>Cerebral palsy</u>, <u>Learning disabilities</u>, <u>Attention-deficit hyperactivity disorder</u>, <u>Autism</u>, <u>Spina bifida</u>, hearing and vision disorders, and <u>Conduct disorders</u>.

Developmental Test. A measure of a child's performance in age-related tasks such as language, perceptual-motor, social, self-care, emotional, and ambulation.

Dexterity. The ability to use the body in a coordinated and purposeful manner. When using the term dexterity, most therapists refer to the ability of the upper extremity to manipulate objects. Dexterity may be subdivided into manual or gross dexterity, which is the movement of the arm and hand to work in larger patterns and with larger objects; and finger or fine dexterity, which is the movement of the fingers in small patterns or with small objects. For similar terms and treatment, see <u>Coordination</u>, <u>Gross motor</u>, and <u>Fine motor</u>.

Diagonal Patterns. Patterns of movement used within Voss' (1967; Voss, Iota, & Myers, 1985) framework of proprioceptive neuromuscular facilitation to help remediate motor control. A flexion and extension component are added together to produce a diagonal movement which imitates movement that occurs during functional activities. See Motor control problems, Proprioceptive neuromuscular facilitation for further discussion of diagonal patterns.

Diathesis. A predisposition or vulnerability to a specific disease, disorder, or condition. A stress-diathesis refers to the precipitating episode of symptoms that leads to a disease through a stressful event or stressors in the environment.

DIP. Distal interphalangeal.

Diplegia. Paralysis of two extremities.

Diplopia. Double vision.

Disability. Any restriction or lack (resulting from an impairment) of ability to perform an activity in the manner or within the range considered normal for a human being. These human activities include walking, running, speaking, writing, dressing, feeding oneself, or listening. A psychiatric or physical disability results from the symptoms of an illness such as Aphasia, Hemiplegia, Dysphagia, Auditory impairment, Delusions or Hallucinations that can prevent an individual from engaging in everyday human activities. For example, the symptoms of Depression can cause an individual to become disabled in working (World Health Organization, 1980).

Discourse Analysis. The study of language as communication through the forms and mechanisms of verbal interaction.

Dislocation. An abnormal separation of bones that limits motions at the joint and therefore prevents functional activity.

Distal. See Anatomical position.

Dopamine. A catecholamine neurotransmitter that occurs naturally in the brain and effects arousal in the autonomic nervous system. An overabundance of dopamine has been implicated as a factor in the etiology of Schizophrenia. A paucity of dopamine is associated with Parkinson's disease and tardive dyskinesia. L-dopa, the precursor of dopamine, is used in the treatment of Parkinson's disease. Medications that block the action of dopamine are used to treat schizophrenia.

Dorsal Splint. A splint that is applied to the dorsal surface of the forearm, hand, and/or fingers. This type of splint may be used as a static application to immobilize the wrist without compressing the carpal tunnel, or as a base for hardware, which will produce a dynamic application to substitute for extensor muscles in the case of extensor tendon repair.

Dorsiflexion. A joint motion at the ankle that results in the toes being pulled upward toward the knee. This is ankle joint extension, which is often mislabeled as flexion. See Appendix E for the normal range of this motion.

Down Syndrome. A type of mental retardation caused by a genetic defect where an extra chromosome (21 or 22) is present at birth. The individual's intellectual potential can range from educable to profound mental retardation. Early sensory stimulation programs, gross motor activities, special education, and vocational preparation are critical aspects of habilitation programs for individuals. Although the main symptom is mental retardation, other associated conditions include heart problems, a flat face, large tongue, and decreased muscle tone. The cause is unknown; however, the age of the person's mother is associated with this condition. Mothers who are 40 years of age or older have a higher incidence of children with Down syndrome.

Specific Treatments
- Provide proper positioning as an infant
- As an infant, complete handling activities for sensory stimulation

- Increase the strength of antigravity muscles to assist with trunk control, posture, ROM, and stability
- Complete activities to increase both gross and fine motor coordination
- Promote the use of both hands and playing at midline for bilateral integration
- Apply different textures to decrease tactile defensiveness and increase sensory stimulation
- Provide proprioceptive stimulation through joint compression, playing "wheelbarrow," bouncing on a ball, or weighted objects
- Increase vestibular stimulation with scooterboard, swing, or rotational devices such as merry-go-round to also help decrease gravitational insecurity
- Provide auditory input
- Complete activities to increase the patient's equilibrium and righting reactions necessary for balance and protection
- Educate the patient or the patient's parents on a home program for follow through
- Complete Self-care activities to increase patient's self-esteem and independence
- Work on oral motor development to increase feeding and dental hygiene ability

Contraindications/Precautions

- Be aware that the occipitoatlantal or atlantoaxial joint (C1–C2 joints) may be at risk for subluxation or displacement
- Watch for ligament laxity
- Spinning or contact sports may be contraindicated
- Be aware that the patient may have heart problems such as congenital heart disease which can affect endurance
- Be prepared since the patient may be at risk for seizures
- Allergies or asthma may also be a risk factor for particular activities

- The patient may also demonstrate ear problems that can affect hearing and/or balance as well as vision problems which can affect function

Down Syndrome

Dream Therapy. A method of using dreams, as in psychoanalysis, to gain access to the unconscious by examining the content of dreams. Using a dream diary is helpful in this process. The use of dreams and the dream state to accomplish physical and emotional healing involves both interpretation and the active participation of the client in the dream process.

Dressing. An activity of daily living (ADL) that is essential to an individual's Self-care. See Self-care for specific adaptive techniques, Assistive technology for adaptive equipment, and specific diagnoses/conditions for further discussion and treatment.

Dressing Apraxia. See Apraxia.

Duchenne's Muscular Dystrophy. A disorder that results in general weakness and wasting of the skeletal muscles that control the pelvis and upper and lower proximal extremities. Persons with this type of muscular dystrophy usually do not live longer than 20–25 years of age. The cause of Duchenne's muscular dystrophy is a sex-linked recessive gene, which is carried on the X chromosome. Eight other types of muscular dystrophy have been identified, including myotonic MD, Becker MD, limb-girdle MD, facioscapulohumeral MD, congenital MD, oculopharyngeal MD, distsal MD, and Emery-Dreifuss MD.

Specific Treatments
- Complete activities to maintain gross motor coordination
- Fabricate splints and recommend positioning devices to prevent deformity
- Maintain the patient's endurance
- Preserve muscle strength, especially at the large joints, which are responsible for ambulation, as well as ROM
- Provide activities to maintain fine motor coordination and dexterity
- Complete activities, such as swimming, to maintain the strength of muscles for respiration

- Educate the patient on work simplification and energy conservation principles
- Recommend power equipment such as power wheelchairs when needed
- Consult the patient and family on diet restrictions to assist the patient with easier chewing and swallowing
- Complete a home evaluation and make recommendations for equipment to increase safety and mobility in the home
- Encourage the patient to attend support group meetings for socialization and emotional adjustment to the disease
- Instruct the patient on assistive devices to increase independence with Self-care activities
- Explore leisure skills to help the patient feel productive

Contraindications/Precautions

- Avoid exposure of the patient with persons who have respiratory infections or colds
- Communicate changes in respiration or signs of respiratory distress to the physician

Dynamic Splint. See Splint.

Dysarthria. Difficulty with the production of speech. A patient who has dysarthria may display slurred speech, a nasal tone, a difference in pitch of voice, or explosive speech. This deficit may result from a cerebellar lesion.

Dysdiadochokinesia. Difficulty in completing quick alternating movements, such as supination/pronation or elbow flexion/extension, in a smooth and rhythmic manner. A complete inability in completing this movement is adiadochokinesia. This deficit results from a cerebellar lesion. Treatment should focus on compensatory techniques to allow the patient to complete necessary functional activities.

Dysmetria. The inability to complete the ROM needed to reach a target. This deficit in coordination displays itself when a patient is asked to touch a target such as the therapist's finger, the patient's own nose, or an object resting on

Dysmetria. *(continued)*
the table. A cerebellar lesion may result in this type of incoordination. Treatment should focus on compensatory techniques to allow the patient to complete necessary functional activities.

Dyssynergia.   The inability to accomplish a smooth and
complete movement. A patient with this deficit will
demonstrate many small and jerky motions rather than one
total movement. This deficit results from a cerebellar
lesion, and treatment should focus on compensatory techniques to allow the patient to complete necessary functional activities.

Dysthymic Disorder.   A chronically depressed mood
occurring over a period of at least 2 years in which the individual experiences the symptoms of depression for most of
the day. See Depression.

Dystonia.   A motor disorder characterized by stiffening in
muscles and sudden contractions or "jerky" movements of
the arms, neck, or face. It involves a peculiar twisting movements of the trunk or proximal musculature, which can
result in odd posture and muscle spasms. This deficit is a
type of Athetosis, and it results from a lesion in the basal
ganglia. It is sometimes a side effect of long-term usage of
antipsychotic drugs. See Coordination for specific treatment suggestions.

Eccentric Contraction. See Contraction.

Edema. When tissue is injured, white blood cells rush to the site of injury to help control infection. This inflammatory response causes swelling, or edema, in and around the affected area. The edema may continue due to damaged structures, immobility, or overuse of the affected limb/area. If the therapist uses modalities that help heat superficial and/or underlying tissues, vasodilation occurs and allows increased blood flow to the area. Healing may be facilitated through increased blood flow, but increased fluid will also surround the area; so edema control techniques should be used following the application of heat. Increased fluid creates resistance, which will prevent movement at a joint or movement of underlying tissues. This fluid also tightens the skin, which makes movement more difficult. If edema is not treated, a fibrous material begins to fill the affected area. This fiber deposits within spaces between structures and reduces the ability of those structures to glide. Scar adhesions may begin to form as well. As the patient decreases use of the edematous area, tissue atrophy begins to occur. Edema must be controlled early in treatment to increase or maintain mobility of the affected limb/area. The therapist should monitor edema through circumferential or volumetric measurements in order to document progress.

Edema Control Techniques

- **Elevation**: The patient should elevate the affected part above the heart to facilitate return of the fluid to the lymph system. For example, a patient who has hemiplegia often demonstrates edema in the affected upper extremity. When the patient is lying in bed, the affected upper extremity should be elevated on pillows. If two pillows are available, one should be placed under the entire forearm with the second placed only under the hand. This creates a better incline for the arm toward the heart. If only one pillow is available, the therapist can place the pillow under the entire forearm and double the distal end of the pillow over itself, so that the pillow beneath the patient's hand is at a greater incline. The patient should also have the upper extremity supported while sitting. If the patient is in a wheelchair, an elevated arm trough, which slides onto the armrest of the wheelchair, can be used. If this special equipment is not available, a pillow can again be propped under the affected extremity. Special inclined cushions can be purchased to place in a nonelevating arm trough, or for use in a hand clinic during treatment.

- **Contrast Baths**: By placing the affected limb in alternating temperatures of water, vasodilation and vasoconstriction occur successively. The action of the blood vessels creates a mechanical pump, which helps push the increased fluid out of the affected area. The recommended temperatures for the water range from 96°–111° F for the warm water, and 36°–65° F for the cold water. Treatment typically begins with a warm water soak for 3 minutes. The patient is then encouraged to immerse the limb in the cold water for 30–60 seconds. Treatment should alternate between the 3-minute warm soaks and 1-minute cold soaks for duration of treatment up to 20–30 minutes. Treatment should conclude with a final soak for 3 minutes in the warm water. This treatment may also be effective with patients who are hypersensitive or those who have reflex sympathetic dystrophy. The cold water immersion may be painful. It is the writer's experience that patients tolerate the treatment better if the therapist immerses one hand as well. The therapist is then able to identify with the patient's discomfort and empathize on a personal level.

Contraindications/Precautions. See Physical agent modalities for general guidelines when using heat and cold. Patients who have small vessel disease from diabetes, Burger's disease, and arteriosclerotic endarteritis should not complete this treatment.

- **Retrograde Massage**: This technique is used for a

patient who has hand, wrist, or forearm edema. The therapist can passively move the fluid toward the heart through massage. The patient should elevate the hand, either on an inclined cushion or simply setting the elbow on a table and holding the hand straight up from the elbow. The therapist should use lotion and apply equal pressure with both hands to either side of the forearm, while slowly and firmly pressing in a proximal direction from the wrist to the elbow. After the forearm looks less swollen (maybe 8–10 strokes), the therapist should massage the palm and dorsal surface of the hand by starting at the MP joints and pushing proximally toward the wrist. Again, the therapist should use both hands while applying equal pressure to either side of the hand. Once the hand demonstrates decreased edema, the therapist should place circumferential pressure around the finger while massaging from the fingertip toward the MP joint. Each finger is massaged individually, and then the therapist can use both hands to apply pressure to dorsal and volar surfaces of the four digits at the same time. The thumb is completed separately. After the fingers show improvement, the therapist should again massage the hand in the above manner. Finally, the forearm should be massaged to force the last of the moveable fluid from the area toward the heart. This method is based on the physical principle that fluid moves from an area of greater concentration toward an area of lesser concentration. Fluid will not be able to move from the fingers to the hand if the hand already has an increased concentration of fluid. However, if the extra fluid is moved from the hand, then the fluid in the fingers will physically *want* to move from the fingers (high concentration) to the hand (lesser concentration). Likewise, if the forearm contains increased fluid, it will not accept more fluid. Therefore, the fluid should first be removed from the forearm, then the hand, and finally the fingers.

However, the fluid from the fingers should not be allowed to remain in the hand, and massage should be completed to force that fluid from the hand to the forearm and then back to the heart.

- **Compression**: The application of snug garments to an edematous extremity also helps push extra fluid from the limb toward the heart. If using a wrap such as Coban, the wrap should begin distally and work proximally to promote flow of the fluid back toward the heart. Care should be taken so that the area is not wrapped too tightly; this may decrease blood flow to the area. A patient with hand and finger edema can wear an Isotoner glove throughout the day. The therapist should use the opposite glove and turn it inside out to apply it to the affected hand. For example, a patient who has hemiplegia may demonstrate edema in the right hand. The therapist would order a left glove and then turn it inside out and place it on the right hand. This prevents the seams of the glove from indenting the edema, and it provides a more uniform pressure to the fingers. Finally, specially ordered garments can be purchased to provide compression to an edematous limb. For example, a patient with breast cancer may demonstrate moderate to severe edema in the entire upper extremity nearest the cancer site. The patient can be measured for a Jobst or other garment, which compresses the entire limb from the wrist to the shoulder. An Isotoner glove then may also be applied to prevent fluid from pooling in the hand.
- **Active Motion**: Movement of the affected area increases blood flow, which helps the removal of extra fluid. The therapist should stress that slight wiggling movements are not beneficial. The patient must complete full ROM, or as close as possible, to receive maximum benefits with edema control.
- **Ice**: Vasoconstriction occurs from the application of cold. When dilated blood vessels at a site of injury are quickly

caused to constrict, a natural pumping effect occurs which helps move extra fluid back toward the heart.

Types of Edema
- **Brawny Edema**: This area of swelling is hard when palpated.
- **Pitting Edema**: On palpation, this type of swelling will be soft and indent with pressure.

Electrical Stimulation. Applying an electrical stimulus to help facilitate muscular control.

Electroencephalograph (EEG). An instrument for detecting and recording the electrical potential produced by the brain cells. Brain-wave activity is recorded indicating alpha, beta, delta, and theta rhythms, which describe the range of cycles per second of the amplitude of the signal. An individual producing alpha waves (8–12 second waves) is usually in a very relaxed state whereas beta waves (15–30 seconds) are indicative of normal consciousness. EEG is used in Biofeedback training.

Electromyograph (EMG). An instrument to record the electrical activity of muscles by applying surface electrodes (transducers) or needle electrodes into the muscle. Along with the EMG, an oscilloscope and amplifier are used in Biofeedback to record muscle activity, for example, the frontalis muscles in Relaxation therapy.

Endorphin. A polypeptide component found naturally in the brain that acts as a natural analgesic by binding to opiate receptor sites. Some researchers have found that endorphins are produced by aerobic exercise such as jogging and fast walking.

Endurance. A musculoskeletal and cardiopulmonary component that enables the individual to engage in a motor activity over time. It is the ability to continue activity for a specific length of time. Treatment plans to increase

Endurance

Endurance. *(continued)*

endurance require prolonged effort in walking, or working in an occupation. Graded activity programs are used to increase endurance.

To continue activity, the muscles cannot contract maximally or the patient would fatigue quickly. The patient uses the muscles for a *moderate* level of activity, and treatment serves to gradually lengthen the time that the patient participates in the activity to help increase the patient's endurance. A patient should take rest breaks as needed, with the goal being that the rest breaks will become shorter in duration and frequency during the treatment session. Below are some activities that can help increase endurance.

Treatment Methods

- Upper extremity bicycle: The bicycle may be set on a lower resistance, but the patient should continue pedaling for a greater length of time than if the patient was using the bicycle for strengthening purposes
- Ring tree: The patient may use one or both extremities to retrieve one ring at a time from a horizontal rod on one side of the "tree" and move it to a horizontal rod on the other side of the "tree"
- Sanding on an inclined surface
- Cooking activity
- Balloon volleyball
- Woodworking: Sanding and putting a birdhouse kit together
- Folding laundry
- Dressing
- Light cleaning activities such as doing the dishes or clearing a table after a meal
- Pulleys: The patient should be given a target time to continue using the pulleys before a rest break may be taken, and emphasis should be placed on continuing movement through full range versus moving the pulleys rapidly

Energy Conservation. A treatment technique that provides the patient with procedures to reduce energy expenditure during activities. First, the patient should be made aware of the energy required for particular activities; if the therapist wishes to be *very* specific, Metabolic equivalent tables may be used to provide the patient with exact amounts of energy required for activities. The patient should then be instructed on principles and techniques that will help the patient conserve energy while completing tasks. This allows the patient a higher quality of life by allowing the patient to maintain independence with a greater number of tasks. If the patient is not aware of these methods, he or she may run out of energy early in the day and require help with any functions throughout the rest of the day. Patients who have cardiac dysfunctions, pulmonary conditions, or poor endurance can benefit from these principles. See Metabolic equivalent for additional information.

Equilibrium Reaction. See Reflexes and reactions.

Ergonomics. The principle of fitting the job or environment to the worker, or homemaker. The occupational therapist using ergonomics considers the tools, equipment, seating, dials, lighting, colors, and placement of furniture, appliances, and other parts of the environment in preventing work injuries, and enhancing function. The physical and psychological characteristics of the individual are considered in devising an environment where the occupational therapist tries to place the worker or homemaker in an anatomically neutral position as well as reducing the stressors.

- *Ergonomic Job Analysis*. An open-ended process that includes a detailed inspection, description; and evaluation of the workplace, equipment, tools, work methods, and the human factors that impact on performing a job (Keyserling, Armstrong, & Punnett, 1991).

- *Risk Factors*. Variables related to performing a job that can potentially lead to injuries, illnesses, or diseases. These factors can include the environment, for example, extreme temperature, poorly designed tools, an uncomfortable chair, work methods such as using poor lifting techniques, undue or continual stress, and repetitive motions.

Ethnoscience.   The study of the characteristics of language as culture in terms of lexical and/or semantic relations.

Etiology.   Examination of the cause or causes of an illness or disease. There are predisposing and precipitating factors that lead to the onset of a disease. Most mental illnesses have multiple risk factors such as genetic, physiological, developmental, psychological, and sociological factors that can predispose a vulnerable individual to mental illness. Stress and sudden losses can precipitate an episode of mental illness in an individual who is vulnerable.

Evaluation.   Analysis of an individual's behavior, characteristics, aptitudes, and present functioning gained through specific tests, clinical observations, and procedures that can be used for treatment planning or discharge recommendations.

Eversion.   See Anatomical position.

Executive Functions of the Brain.   Higher level cognitive tasks such as abstraction, sequential organization, motor planning, and decision making.

Exercise.   See Prescribed exercise.

Expressed Emotion (EE).   A concept related to a family's psychological interactions with a family member who is mentally ill (e.g., has a diagnosis of schizophrenia). The criteria for high expressed emotion are based on factors such as negative comments about family member, personal criticism, dissatisfaction with individual's behavior, lack of warmth expressed toward individual, and constant worry about individual. An indication of high expressed emotion toward a family member with mental illness has been linked to a higher relapse rate in individuals with schizophrenia living in the community than those individuals living in household with low expressed emotion (Brown, Birley, & Wing, 1972).

Extension.   See <u>Anatomical position</u>.

Extensor Synergy.   An automatic pattern of movement that may occur when a patient with hemiplegia attempts the motion of extension, such as elbow or knee extension. The stereotypical pattern for the upper extremity combines the following motions: scapular abduction and depression, shoulder adduction and internal rotation, elbow extension, forearm pronation, wrist and finger extension. The stereotypical pattern for the upper extremity combines the following motions: hip adduction, extension, and internal rotation; knee extension; ankle plantar flexion and inversion; and toe flexion. See <u>Motor control problems</u>, <u>Movement therapy of Brunnstrom</u> for treatment methods.

Extensor Thrust (Reflex).   See <u>Reflexes and reactions</u>.

External.   See <u>Anatomical position</u>.

External Rotation.   See <u>Anatomical position.</u>

Extinction.   Elimination or inhibition of behavior by not reinforcing behavior.

Facilitation. The act of increasing or supporting. Often used when referring to a patient who demonstrates low muscle tone. See Motor control problems for applications of facilitation.

Facilitation Techniques. Techniques, which help, increase the tone of a muscle so that it is able to contract and cause movement. Some examples include Brushing, Stroking, Tapping, and Vibration. See Motor control problems for more examples.

Family Therapy. Process of treating an individual by focusing on the dynamics in the family. In this process, the communication patterns of the family are emphasized as well as the relationships between family members. Therapists try to assist the family by providing insight into the dynamics of interactions and by helping family members to develop healthy and honest communication. Role playing can be used in facilitating this process.

Feeding/Eating. An activity of daily living (ADL) that is essential to an individual's Self-care. See Self-care for specific adaptive techniques, Assistive technology for adaptive equipment, and specific diagnoses/conditions for further discussion and treatment.

Feldenkrais Method A motor therapy that involves learning new patterns of movement to enhance the communication between the brain and body. The method includes lying on one's back, sitting, or standing while becoming aware of each movement. The therapist or instructor may use massage to reduce stress or muscular tension. The purposes of this method are to reduce joint pain, improve joint mobility, increase muscle coordination, and improve posture.

Forensic Psychiatry. The application of psychiatry and psychosocial practice to individuals who have committed a crime or are incarcerated for an illegal offense. In 1999, approximately 5.3 million individuals were incarcerated in penal institutions or on probation for a convicted crime. Occupational therapists working in correctional institutions, psychiatric intensive care units in prisons, or community facilities for individuals on probation employ various activities to engage the individual in everyday occupations. The purposes of these programs are to foster community living skills such as in preparation for Work, literacy, social skills, communication, Stress management, and anger management. The overall purposes of these programs are to promote self-worth, individual responsibility, and self-regulation. Individual and group therapy techniques are employed to achieve these goals.

Festinating Gait. Gait that is characterized by small, shuffling steps, which propel the patient's body forward in an increasing rate. Patients who have a lesion in the substantia nigra often demonstrate this deficit. See Parkinson's disease for treatment and further discussion.

Fetal Alcohol Syndrome (FAS). A disability including intellectual and learning deficits, ADHD, and deficient growth patterns. Caused by intake of alcohol by the mother during pregnancy. Facial characteristics include small head, eyes, and jaws; a wide, flat nose bridge; and lack of a groove between the lip and the nose.

Figure/Ground Perception. The ability to discriminate between an object and its background. For instance, a patient who has difficulty with figure/ground perception may be unable to find a white piece of paper lying on top of a white bedsheet. See Cognitive-perceptual deficits for further discussion and treatment.

Fine Motor Coordination. The ability to control the contraction of small muscles to complete fine, precise movements. Examples of functional activities using fine motor skills are crocheting, tying shoelaces, opening up a

Fine Motor Coordination. *(continued)*
can, and handwriting. See Coordination for treatment
methods.

Finger Agnosia.   The inability to name or identify a specific finger when asked to discriminate between fingers,
usually during a sensory evaluation. See Cognitive-perceptual deficits for further discussion and treatment

Finger Extension.   See Reflexes and reactions.

Flaccidity.   A decrease in Muscle tone, also referred to as
Hypotonicity and most often present immediately following a stroke. The patient should have a large range of
motion available passively; however, very little, if any,
active motion can be observed. The patient may be at danger for Subluxation of the head of the humerus if the low
muscle tone continues for any length of time. See Motor
control problems and Cerebral vascular accident (CVA) for
treatment methods.

Flashback.   Recurrence of a traumatic event, memory
trace, emotion, or perceptual experience. It is present in
individuals with Post-traumatic stress disorders.

Flat Affect.   See Affect.

Flexion.   See Anatomical position.

Flexor Synergy.   An automatic pattern of movement that
may occur when a patient with hemiplegia attempts the
motion of flexion, such as elbow or knee flexion. The
stereotypical pattern for the upper extremity combines the
following motions: scapula adduction and elevation, shoulder abduction and external rotation, elbow flexion, forearm
supination, wrist and finger flexion. The stereotypical pattern for the lower extremity combines the following
motions: hip flexion, abduction, and external rotation; knee

flexion; ankle dorsiflexion and inversion, and toe extension. See <u>Motor control problems</u>, <u>Movement therapy of Brunnstrom</u> for treatment methods.

Flexor Withdrawal. See <u>Reflexes and reactions</u>.

Fluidotherapy. The application of a dry heat modality consisting of cellulose particles held in a container and moved in air. The turbulence of the mixture generates a thermal effect when objects are immersed in the medium. It uses convection to transfer heat to superficial physiological tissues. See <u>Physical agent modalities</u> for further discussion and treatment.

Form constancy. The perceptual process of being able to recognize an object in various positions, sizes, and environments. Reading letters and numbers and identifying objects depend on this skill. This process is also dependent upon <u>Object permanence</u>.

Fragile X Syndrome. A male with this syndrome has an X chromosome which has a weak area on the long arm of the X. This weak area often results in the end of the long arm separating from the rest of the chromosome. Persons with this diagnosis demonstrate mental retardation. Fragile X is the second leading cause of mental retardation that can be diagnosed from a specific cause.

Frame of Reference. Based on a theoretical model or theory that generates specific evaluation and treatment techniques in clinical practice. Psychodynamic, model of human occupation, cognitive-behavioral, and sensory integration are frames of reference in psychosocial occupational therapy. Other frames of references in occupational therapy include neurodevelopmental, cognitive-disabilities, occupational adaptation, ecology of human performance, biomechanical, and motor learning.

Framework for Support (Trainor & Church, 1984). A conceptual model based on self-help; family, friends, and neighbors; community resources; and the formal mental health system. An important premise of this approach is that individuals with mental health problems should be empowered to control their own lives (Carling, 1995).

Friction massage.   See Massage.

Functional.   The degree of a client's independence in the performance areas of Work/productivity and Leisure.

Functional Capacity Assessment (FCA).   Comprehensive and systematic approach that measures the client's overall physical ability such as muscle strength, endurance, joint range of motion, ambulation, sitting, standing, and lifting related to work activities. Examples of FCAs are *Isernhagen Work System Functional Capacity Evaluation Procedures, Baltimore Therapeutic Equipment, Key Functional Capacity Assessment,* and *Blankenship System.*

Functional Electrical Stimulation (FES).   A term used for Neuromuscular electrical stimulation (NMES) while applying the current to a patient during the attempt of functional activities. See Physical agent modalities for further discussion and treatment of NMES.

Functional Position.   A position that allows a person to complete necessary functional activities, even if that position is fixed so that movement is limited to that single position. See Functional position of the hand.

Functional Position of the Hand.   If Contractures are unavoidable, a patient should be positioned so that he or she has some functional use of the hand, even though the hand has limited ROM. The most functional position of the hand is slight wrist extension (10° to 30°) with thumb abduction and slight flexion, and finger flexion through partial ROM (Zemke, 1995). If the hand contracts while fully flexed or extended, the patient will not be able to use the hand for any activities. If the hand contracts in this partially flexed position, then the patient has the opportunity to use the hand to hold or stabilize items or assist with functional activities such as dressing. The position of the hand that provides optimal length of the intrinsic muscles (also referred to Intrinsic-plus position) is another recommended position for immobilization (James, 1970). In this position, the MP joints are flexed to near 90° while the PIP and DIP joints are fully extended. This helps prevent atrophy of the intrinsic muscles, which would cause the patient to lose the ability to cup the palm/hand. If a patient has some shortening of the muscles and is not able to compositely flex at the MP, PIP, and DIP joints through partial ROM, this position may be more achievable since flexion is occurring only at the MP joints in this position.

Galvanic Skin Response (GSR). The change in the electrical resistance of the skin reflecting the individual's emotional state. What is being measured is the conductive pathway of a sweat gland, which is associated with an individual's sympathetic response. The GSR is traditionally used in "lie detector" tests.

General Systems Theory. A model of understanding the relationships between people and organizations and between parts and wholes (von Bertalanffy, 1950).

Generalization. A cognitive ability to apply learned concepts and behaviors to new situations such as using tools, driving different cars, adapting to social situations, and engaging in a sport. Generalization is important in applying basic skills in Self-care, Leisure, and Work activities.

Gestalt Therapy. A form of humanistic psychotherapy developed by Perls (1969) that emphasizes the client's awareness of the perceptual environment and the "here and now." It utilizes self-awareness exercises to teach the client to be sensitive to the sensory stimuli in the environment.

Global Aphasia. See Aphasia.

Global Assessment of Function (GAF) Scale. Grades a client's functioning on a scale of 1 to 100, with 1 indicating that the client is a persistent danger to self or others and a rating of 100 indicating that an individual is functioning at a superior level in a wide range of activities, has many positive qualities, and no symptoms. The scale is based on a mental health-mental illness continuum (APA, 1994).

Goal Attainment Scaling (GAS). An evaluation tool used to describe the personal goals of clients on five possible levels of outcome for each goal. For example, a client can identify lack of assertiveness as a personal problem. A therapeutic strategy is implemented to help the client to improve (Ottenbacher & Cusick, 1989).

Graphesthesia.   The ability to identify numbers, letters, or symbols traced on the skin with vision blocked. Asking the patient to report which items are traced on the patient's palm or fingertips with a dull pencil or instrument while blocking the patient's vision can test this perceptual skill.

Grasp.   The act of positioning the hand so that objects are held against the palm and the palmar surface of the fingers. Most grasp patterns include the thumb in opposition to help complete this task. When a patient with Hemiplegia is just beginning to regain hand motion, grasp is sometimes referred to as mass or gross grasp since a specific pattern is not seen. Rather, the patient is simply beginning to flex the fingers in order to hold objects. Specific grasp patterns which can be observed in patients with normal muscle tone and coordination include:

Types of Grasp

- **Cylindrical Grasp**: Grasp that uses the thumb to oppose against a cylindrical object so that the object is held against the palm and palmar surface of the fingers. The fingers flex and each joint to curve around the sur-face of the object being held. This grasp is used when holding a soda can or handle of a hammer.

- **Spherical Grasp**: Grasp that uses the thumb to oppose against a round object to hold it against the palm and pal-mar surface of the fingers. This grasp differs from the cylin-drical grasp since the ring and small fingers flex more around a round object, which helps to cup the palm. This grasp is used when holding a baseball or apple.

- **Hook Grasp**: Grasp with the fingers that does not include the thumb. The MCP joints of the fingers are extended (or may be hyperextended) while the PIP and DIP joints are flexed. This grasp is used when holding the handle of a suitcase or briefcase. This hand position may also be observed following nerve damage to the upper extremity or during the return of muscle tone to the upper extremity after a stroke.

Grasp

Grasp

- **Intrinsic Plus Grasp**: Grasp that uses the thumb to oppose near the ring and small fingers to help hold an object against the palm and palmar surface of the fingers. All fingers flex at the MP joint while fully extending at the PIP and DIP joints. This grasp is used when holding a plate or book.

Grasp Reflex.   See Reflexes and reactions.

Grooming.   An activity of daily living (ADL) essential to an individual's Self-care. See Self-care for specific adaptive techniques, Assistive technology for adaptive equipment, and specific diagnoses/conditions for further discussion and treatment.

Gross Motor Coordination.   The ability to control the contraction of large muscles and groups of muscles to complete large, less specific movements when engaging in everyday activities such as walking, running, bicycling, and in sports such as swimming, tennis, and basketball. See Coordination, Range of motion treatment methods.

Group Dynamics.   The study of the factors and conditions that affect the actions in a group, for example, the building of group cohesion and leadership functions.

Group Therapy.   The applications of group methods to help clients gain insight, learn skills, prepare for employment, express feelings, and try out new behaviors. It is appropriate with almost all clients including those with psychosocial and physical disabilities, and cognitive deficits. The therapist should consider the following factors in establishing a group:
- Group goals are identified by therapist and clients, such as stress management, prevocational preparation, creative expression, pain management, and prevention of work injuries.

- Structure for group is established considering the number of clients in group, number of sessions, length of each session, and area where group will take place.
- Administrative contract is established where the therapist gains the approval for group from administrator and inter-disciplinary team.
- Clients are selected for group considering age, gender, diagnosis individual treatment goals and client motivation to be in group.
- Therapeutic leadership style is considered such as democratic, therapist-controlled, or leaderless group.
- Group methodology is designed considering use of lectures, seminar, Role playing, video taping, and demonstrations.
- Media and modalities used in group are selected such as arts and crafts, dance, music, poetry, cooking, computers, prevocational tests.
- The effectiveness of group is determined through psychometrics, self-reports, family and staff clinical observations.

Occupational therapists have traditionally run groups in social skills, stress management, creative arts and leisure activities, anger management, assertiveness training, employment preparation, and dealt with self-care issues as in arthritis, stroke and low back pain.

Guiding.   A treatment technique used by Bobath to help a patient relearn normal movement while the therapist places his or her hand on the patient's arm and helps move it through patterns. See Motor control problems, Neurodevelopmental approach.

Guillain-Barré Syndrome.   A condition that causes demyelination of peripheral nerves and results in muscle weakness and sensory loss. Hemiplegia and Hemiparesis occur in an ascending manner, but remyelination often occurs, which causes the condition to descend. The onset

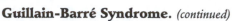

Guillain-Barré Syndrome. *(continued)*

lasts for 1–3 weeks, followed by a plateau period when no change occurs, followed by remyelination, which can take up to 2 years. The cause is unknown, but a virus may be responsible for the attack of peripheral nerves by the immune system.

Specific Treatments

- Maintain ROM, both passively and actively, as paralysis descends
- Utilize nonresistive activities for strengthening until patient is able to demonstrate muscle strength of 3/5 (see Manual muscle test), then patient may begin gentle and graded resistive activity
- Fabricate splints to prevent deformity from atrophy of muscles
- Complete activities for bilateral integration and coordination
- Increase endurance by slowly increasing time during which the patient participates in therapy
- Provide sensory stimulation as the sensation returns
- Educate the patient on progression of the disease and expectations for treatment
- Instruct the patient on principles of energy conservation and work simplification
- Teach joint protection principles
- Train the patient to use Stress management and Relaxation therapy as needed
- Stress the importance of avoiding fatigue as it may trigger a setback in recovery
- Encourage the patient to join a support group for socialization and adjustment to the disease
- Retrain Self-care activities using compensatory techniques and assistive devices as needed
- Complete a home and/or job site evaluation and provide recommendations to modify the environment for increased independence with activities

- Explore new leisure interests as needed

Contraindications/Precautions

- Monitor the skin for redness over bony prominences, which could result in pressure sores
- Discontinue activity if the patient becomes fatigued
- Prevent substitution of muscles that are not the prime movers for a motion during strengthening or ROM
- Provide equipment to maintain proper positioning
- Stop at the point of pain when completing PROM

Gustatory Sensation. Receiving, discriminating, localizing, and interpreting taste mainly through the receptors on the tongue.

Guillain-Barré Syndrome

Habilitation. The development of function in the performances of work, leisure, and self-care by an individual with a developmental disability such as <u>Autism</u> or <u>Cerebral palsy</u>. In some cases adults with chronic mental illness who have not developed functional abilities are taught these competencies for the first time and are considered to be habilitated rather than rehabilitated.

Habituation. Refers to the daily adaptive behavior or routines of an individual as described in the <u>Model of Human Occupation</u>.

Halfway House. A supportive housing environment in which clients are provided a structured and supportive setting. Frequently clients are given communal responsibilities for maintenance and kitchen tasks. Its purpose is to provide a transition from a hospital to independent living in the community.

Hallucination. A false perception such as seeing, hearing, or smelling a sensation that does not exist in reality. The individual with a hallucination is unable to distinguish between the real and the imagined sensation.

Handicap. A disadvantage for an individual, resulting from an impairment or a disability that limits or prevents the fulfillment of a normal role depending on age, sex, social, and cultural factors. A psychiatric handicap is the inability to perform normal role functions as a student, worker, husband, wife, father, or mother or to engage in <u>Work</u>, <u>Leisure</u> activities, or be independent in <u>Self-care</u> or social functioning. The handicap can also be aggravated by environmental factors such as stigma, which produces a negative attitude toward individuals with mental illness and thereby prevents the individual from obtaining employment (World Health Organization, 1980).

Hand Injuries. The treatment of hand injuries is very specific and specialized; therefore, hand injuries are briefly discussed. For more specific protocol, the therapist may refer to various references including the *Indiana Hand Center Protocol* or the two-volume set, *Rehabilitation of the Hand*. The therapist should take *extreme caution* to talk to the physician for his or her preferred protocol or plan of treatment, since physicians and treatment protocols vary in their approaches to rehabilitation. Some approaches tend to be more conservative, while others are aggressive. The therapist should also consult the physician about precautions and contraindications to treatment; however, many protocols and more-detailed hand references are specific with treatment to prevent injury during the healing process. *Please remember when reading the following material, that this is a general treatment guide for hand therapy which was taken from only a few references since so many varying protocols exist. Please consult further resources when treating specific injuries.*

Types of Injuries

- **Joint Injuries**: Treatment should stress gentle exercise within the patient's tolerance of pain. Exercise should not increase pain or edema; however, if Edema does occur, ice massage or Coban wrapping may help decrease swelling. The therapist should be careful to prescribe exercise for the unaffected part of the hand and the upper extremity to help decrease the loss of function due to weakness or stiffness which may occur while the joint heals.

- **Ligamentous Injuries**: The most common type of this injury affects the proximal interphalangeal (PIP) joint. Treatment should first immobilize the joint with a splint to hold the joint in 15°–20° of flexion for 10–14 days. Immobilization may be required for up to three weeks if instability is noted following the initial 10–14 days of splinting. After the splint is removed, the affected finger may be taped to an adjacent finger to help protect the affected joint while it continues to strengthen.

- **Volar Plate Injuries**: This type of injury is usually caused by hyperextension at a joint. If the injury is not treated properly, the joint may heal with a <u>Swan neck deformity</u>. The affected finger should be immobilized with a splint to hold the joint in 20° of flexion for two weeks. Next, a dorsal blocking splint should be fabricated and worn by the patient for 1–2 more weeks to prevent full extension of the weak joint.

- **Dislocations**: The joint most commonly dislocated is the proximal interphalangeal (PIP) joint. A dislocation that results in a volar plate injury should be treated in the manner listed above. If the proximal interphalangeal joint is dislocated in flexion, then the joint should be splinted in extension. An injury of this type often requires surgical intervention.

Handling. Within the framework of NDT, refers to the therapist's use of his or her hands to assist the patient with movement patterns. When necessary, the therapist facilitates active movement or tone, inhibits abnormal movement or tone, reeducates muscles to complete normal movement patterns, and realigns joints. See <u>Motor control problems</u>, <u>Neurodevelopmental treatment</u> for more treatment techniques.

Health Maintenance Organization (HMO). A prepaid group health care program that provides diagnostic treatment services, ambulatory care, hospitalization, and surgery with an emphasis on prevention.

Hemianesthesia. A complete loss of sensation to either the right or left side of the body.

Hemianopsia. A condition in which a patient is blind in half of the visual field of one or both eyes. If the patient has had a CVA in the occipital lobe, it can result in a *homonymous hemianopsia*, the patient is blind in the corresponding fields in both eyes. For example, a patient who has a left homonymous hemianopsia is blind in the left half of the visual field with both eyes; so the left eye cannot see to the far left, and the right eye cannot see to its left, which would include the area slightly to the left and center of the patient. See Cognitive-perceptual deficits, Visual foundation skills for treatment of visual deficits.

Hemiballism.   Involuntary movement that occurs as rapid gross motor movements which are violent and forceful. The extremities display this deficit as flinging movements, usually on only one side of the body. Lesions of the subthalamic nucleus may result in hemiballism.

Hemiparesis.   Weakness of half of the body, usually resulting from an insult to the brain.

Hemiplegia.   Paralysis of one side of the body, which usually occurs following an insult to the brain.

Herbal/botanical.   A method of using forms of plants for prevention and treatment of illnesses.

Heterotopic Ossification.   The formation of bone in locations where bone does not normally form, such as soft tissue surrounding a joint. Symptoms that may signal ossification include localized pain, redness or warmth, edema, and rapidly decreasing ROM at a joint. Joints, which seem to be at higher risk of involvement include the shoulder, elbow, hip, and knee.
Treatment
- Include AROM throughout the available range, positioning and splinting, or PROM *only* to the point of pain.

- Surgery may be necessary to free a joint and increase ROM.

- Patients who may be at increased risk of heterotopic ossification are those with burns, traumatic brain injury, or spinal cord injury.

High-Voltage Galvanic Stimulation (HVGS). A physical agent modality which uses electrical current to treat pain and edema, improve circulation, reeducate muscles, reduce muscle guarding, decrease atrophy/increase strength, or heal wounds. See Physical agent modalities for further discussion and treatment.

High-Voltage Pulsed Current (HVPC). This modality may also be referred to as high voltage galvanic stimulation (HVGS). See Physical agent modalities for further discussion.

Hippotherapy. Treatment with the help of the horse to strengthen, stretch, and relax the muscles, enhance the motor coordination of the rider, improve posture and attain psychological goals such as increased self-esteem, body image, and self-concept. The rationale for its use as a therapeutic modality is that the horse's movement produces a smooth, rhythmical pattern to the rider. Therapeutic riding programs have been used successfully with clients having diagnoses such as multiple sclerosis, traumatic brain injuries, stroke, learning disabilities, orthopedic disorders, spina bifida, Mental retardation, juvenile delinquency, Cerebral palsy, Autism, and other mental illnesses.

Histrionic Personality Disorder. Characteristic of individuals who are prone to exaggerate, act out or demonstrate feelings, and show explosive personality reactions. In this disorder the individual strives for excitement and surprise in relationships with others. Others characterize individuals as vain, self-centered, demanding, and shallow.

Holistic Medicine. A comprehensive approach to treatment considering the physical, social, psychological, spiritual, and economic needs of the client. Holistic methods include diet therapy, exercise, Stress management, and Relaxation therapy as well as traditional treatments.

Home Evaluation.   Prior to a patient's discharge from the hospital to home, an occupational therapist should evaluate the patient's home to provide recommendations for equipment to be installed and adaptations to be completed. When possible, the physical therapist should accompany the occupational therapist so that all areas are addressed. The patient and a caregiver, when applicable, should accompany the therapists. The patient can demonstrate transfer/mobility and other Self-care activities to show the therapist if the current environment is acceptable. The therapist can also ask the patient and caregiver what the routine was prior to the injury and what the expectations are for routine when the patient returns home. While demonstrating ambulation or transfers, the caregiver can be given recommendations to assist the patient if needed. The therapist should take a tape measure along to measure width of doorways, height of chairs and bed, height of stairs, and so on. The therapist should give recommendations to simplify tasks, remove obstacles, or widen pathways throughout the home. After the evaluation is completed, the therapist should sit down with the patient and caregiver to discuss the results. A list of problem areas, adaptations to solve those problems, and recommendations for equipment to increase the patient's independence should be given to the patient and caregiver. Below is a list of areas that should be assessed during the home evaluation.

Components of the Home Evaluation
- The patient's mobility status and devices used (wheelchair, quad cane, etc.)
- Type of home and number of levels within home, including basement when applicable
- Access from the driveway and/or the garage to the house
- Number of steps at entrance to home, the steps' dimensions, and if railing is installed
- Ramp location and dimensions if applicable
- Size of the threshold at the entrance

- Size of door at entrance and the direction it opens
- Type of floor covering in rooms used by the patient
- If living room arrangement conducive to patient's mobility status
- Height and firmness of furniture used by patient
- Dimensions of hallways and if sharp turns are necessary when entering various rooms
- Door dimensions of bedroom and direction it opens, including threshold height
- Type and height of bed, including patient's ability to transfer to/from bed
- Space in bedroom, including room for wheelchair or hospital bed if needed
- Accessibility of dressers and closet
- Door dimensions of bathroom and direction it opens, including threshold height
- Dimensions of tub, type of water barrier (curtain vs. glass doors), and if shower head available
- Dimensions of door and height of threshold if walk-in shower
- Height of sink and type of faucets
- Height of toilet, toilet paper location, or location near cabinet-type sink to assist patient with standing, including patient's ability to transfer
- Availability for grab bar installation if not currently installed
- Door dimensions of kitchen and direction it opens, including threshold height
- Height of stove, location of oven, location of controls, and accessibility
- Height of sink, type of faucets, and availability for wheelchair to fit beneath if applicable
- Accessibility, type, and location of cupboards
- Accessibility and location of hinge on refrigerator
- Accessibility and locations of necessary switches and outlets

- Height of kitchen table and countertops
- Door dimensions of laundry room and direction it opens, including threshold height
- Dimensions and number of steps to laundry facilities
- Accessibility and type of washer
- Accessibility and type of dryer
- Location of any throw rugs
- Location of phone
- If patient has an emergency call system or list of emergency numbers
- Location of mailbox
- Location of thermostat
- Notation of any unsafe situations like sharp-edged furniture, noninsulated hot water pipes, or imperfect floors
- Notation of cluttered areas
- If patient has a fire extinguisher and its location
- List of equipment the patient currently has
- List of problem situations and areas to be rectified
- Recommendations for adaptations to be made
- Recommendations for equipment to be purchased

Homeopathy. A school of medicine, founded by Dr. S. C. F. Hahnemann in the late 18th century, based on the theory that large doses of drugs that produce symptoms of a disease in healthy people will cure the same symptoms when administered in very small amounts. This is loosely based on the theory that "like cures like." Homeopathic physicians use natural remedies of specially prepared plants and minerals to boost the body's defense mechanisms and healing processes.

Homeostasis. Refers to the state of dynamic equilibrium that internal body organisms strive to maintain through feedback mechanisms and regulatory functions. Cannon (1932) described the processes in the body in maintaining normal values such as heart rate, blood pressure, salt, water, blood sugar, and hemoglobin. Homeostasis also

Home Evaluation

Homeostasis. *(continued)*
refers to the body's reaction to disease such as T-cell production to fight infection.

Homogeneous. Refers to like characteristics such as age, gender, or intelligence.

Homolateral Limb Synkinesis. Demonstration of the same motion in both affected extremities. For example, if the patient tries to flex the affected upper extremity, then the lower extremity also involuntarily flexes. See Motor control problems, Movement therapy of Brunnstrom.

Hook Grasp. See Grasp.

Horizontal Abduction. See Anatomical position.

Horizontal Adduction. See Anatomical position.

Horizontal Plane. See Anatomical position.

Horticulture. The science and art of gardening and cultivating fruits, vegetables, flowers, and plants. Horticulture is used as a therapeutic modality.

Hot Packs. A physical agent modality, which uses conduction to transfer heat to superficial physiological tissue. See Physical agent modalities for further discussion and treatment.

Humanism. A system of beliefs and a theory of knowledge that emphasizes the acceptance of diverse cultural values, capacities, and achievements of human beings. In treatment, it represents the unconditional acceptance of the individual, even when a behavior is unacceptable. It is also related to the humane treatment of individuals with mental illness during the 19th century termed Moral treatment.

Humanitarianism. The promotion of social betterment through social action groups that provide aid, welfare, and opportunities to those in poverty or survivors of wars and natural disasters.

Humor.   Any communication that leads to laughing, smiling, or a feeling of amusement by any of the interacting parties. Humor can be used as a stress reducing method in treatment. There is some evidence that humor stimulates neuropeptides and endorphins that can relieve pain.

Huntington's Chorea.   A condition that results in irregular and involuntary movements of the trunk and limbs that results from degeneration of the basal ganglia. This type of chorea is hereditary.

Hydrotherapy.   A physical agent modality that uses the motion of water and convection to transfer heat to superficial physiological tissue and the physical properties of water to benefit treatment in many ways (Walsh, 1990). Can be used in treating individuals with pain, increasing Range of motion, decreasing stress, enabling exercise, and increasing blood circulation. See Aquatic therapy and Physical agent modalities for further discussion and treatment.

Hyperextension.   A joint motion, which may or may not be beyond the normal range of joint motion in extension, but it is beyond the normal alignment of the body parts. For example, some hyperextension can occur within the curvatures of the spine (lordosis or kyphosis), which would be greater than the normal alignment of the spine but would not be beyond the normal range of motion available in the spine.

Hypersensitivity.   A condition in which normal stimuli cause pain or discomfort. A patient who has had a crushing injury, nerve injury, burn, or other injury may be vulnerable to this condition. The patient often guards the extremity to protect it from painful situations; however, this causes decreased use of the extremity, which leads to impaired function. A patient with this condition should be treated through Desensitization.

Hypertonicity.   Muscle tone that is greater than normal tone and inhibits the patient from completing voluntary

Hypertonicity. *(continued)*
movements. Also referred to as Spasticity, hypertonicity can occur in patients with various Upper motor neuron disorders including Parkinson's disease, Multiple sclerosis, Traumatic brain injury, Spinal cord injury, Cerebral vascular accident, Cerebral palsy, or brain tumors. An increase in Deep tendon reflexes as well as a demonstration of Clonus helps determine a diagnosis of hypertonicity. Hypertonicity can be graded on the following scale:

Grades of Hypertonicity

- **Severe**: presence of a strong Stretch reflex and *strong* resistance to PROM (PROM may not be possible) as well as possible presence of clonus
- **Moderate**: visible stretch reflex and PROM is possible but slow
- **Minimal**: stretch reflex can be palpated but very little resistance to PROM (if any), and AROM may be possible with movement against the spastic muscles slower than normal.

Inhibition techniques may help decrease the muscle tone and make movement easier. See Motor control problems and Cerebral vascular accident (CVA) as well as other cross-referenced disorders listed above for treatment methods.

Hypnotherapy. Treatment by inducing an alternate state of consciousness in which the individual feels relaxed and with little pain. Has been used successfully in some cases to decrease smoking, for obesity and in substance abuse.

Hypothalamic-Pituitary-Adrenocortical Axis. Refers to the complex interactions that occur in the autonomic nervous system that involve neurotransmitters and hormonal secretions. It plays an important role in the stress reaction and in maintaining the health of the individual in homeostatic reactions.

Hypothesis. A statement that predicts results and is testable. An example of a hypothesis is aerobic exercise lower blood pressure in middle-aged sedentary males.

Hypotonicity.   Muscle tone that is less than normal tone and inhibits the patient from completing voluntary movements. Also referred to as Flaccidity, hypotonicity often occurs in patients who have suffered a Stroke/CVA, Facilitation techniques may help increase muscle tone and produce a contraction so that movement is possible. See Motor control problems and Cerebral vascular accident (CVA) for treatment methods.

Icing.   A method used to facilitate Muscle tone. Icing should be done in 3 quick strokes.

Precautions
- Icing should not be completed along the patient's midline, especially to patients with spinal cord injuries at level C4–C5 as this may result in Autonomic dysreflexia.
- Icing should also not be applied above the patient's neck to the trigeminal nerve area (except if using ice in the mouth), to the pinna of the ear, or behind the ear.
- Ice, which is applied to the left shoulder, may cause heart arhythmia or angina, so this technique should not be used when working with patients who have cardiovascular problems.

See Motor control problems, Rood approach for more discussion of Facilitation techniques.

Ideational apraxia.   See Apraxia.

Ideomotor apraxia.   See Apraxia.

Imagery.   Arelaxation technique that involves visualizing relaxing scenes with eyes closed. Many practitioners recommend that the client rotate his or her eyes inward and upward as a warm-up technique before visualizing colors, objects, abstract ideas, and significant people in one's life.

Imitation Synkinesis.   Completing a desired movement with the unaffected extremity while trying to complete that same movement with the affected extremity as a means of facilitation. For example, if the patient is trying to flex the affected shoulder, then he or she will flex the unaffected shoulder simultaneously. Brunnstrom (1970, 1996) created this treatment technique.

Impairment.   Any loss or abnormality of physiological, psychological, or anatomical structure or function such as blindness, deafness, astereognosis, mental retardation, or lack of pain sensation. A psychiatric impairment is, for example, a Delusion, Hallucination, severe Anxiety, phobia, Depression, or any other symptom that interferes with carrying out normal human activities (World Health Organization, 1980).

Incoherence. Incomprehensible speech or thinking.

Independent Living Evaluation. Assessment tools used to measure a client's ability to perform the activities of daily living. An example is the *Barthel Self-care Index*.

Inferior. See Anatomical position.

Inhibition. The act of decreasing or suppressing. Often used when referring to a patient who has high Muscle tone. See Motor control problems for applications of inhibition.

Inhibition Techniques. Techniques that decrease the tone of a muscle so that the distal attachment of the muscle and its body part are able to move in the opposite direction. For example, the goal of inhibition to high tone in the biceps is the extension of the elbow (forearm is the distal attachment of the biceps and extension is the opposite action/direction of the biceps). Inhibition is used to help a spastic muscle relax so that the antagonistic muscle can complete its action as well. Techniques that help decrease high tone include pressure, rocking, and rolling. See Motor control problems for more examples.

Initiation of an Activity. The cognitive ability to begin an activity on one's own. This can become impaired in clients who are depressed, have severe mental retardation, and in individuals with brain damage. Therapists can help clients to initiate an activity by using forward or backward Chaining. This enables the client to complete or participate in the activity such as in dressing.

Innate Intelligence. The inherited biological aptitudes and abilities of an individual.

Instinctive Avoiding Reaction. A forward or upward movement of a patient's affected arm results in the involuntary extension and/or hyperextension of the patient's fingers and thumb. See Motor control problems, Movement therapy of Brunnstrom.

Instinctive Grasp Reaction. Similar to the Grasp reflex, the patient's affected hand flexes or closes involuntarily when it comes into contact with a *stationary object*. The patient will not be able to actively extend his or her fingers in order to release the object on command. See Motor control problems, Movement therapy of Brunnstrom.

Institutionalization. An insidious process where, over many years, an individual living in an institution, for example, a state mental hospital, develops apathy, flattened affect, hopelessness, dilapidated appearance, and dependency on others for carrying out activities of daily living.

Instrumental Activities of Daily Living (IADLs). Tasks that involve participation of a client with the physical and/or social environment, including home management, money management, communication, safety, community living skills, work and leisure activities. See Assistive technology and specific diagnoses/conditions for further discussion and treatment.

Intention Tremor. A patient with this deficit demonstrates small involuntary rhythmic movements at one or more joints when attempting voluntary movement. While the patient is at rest, tremors will decrease or may disappear. Once the patient attempts movement, tremors will reappear and may hinder the patient's ability to complete the desired tasks. This deficit results from a cerebellar lesion, and patients who have Multiple Sclerosis often demonstrate intention tremors. See Multiple sclerosis for treatment and further discussion.

Interdisciplinary Team.   Individuals from different disciplines who work cooperatively in generating treatment goals in collaboration with the client.

Interests.   Psychological components that include an individual's choice in engaging in activities such as sports, reading, music, films, theater, arts and crafts, cuisine, and table games. The motivation to engage in activities depend upon the opportunities available to the individual, ability to do the activity, and the pleasure related to the activity. Occupational therapists can help clients to widen their repertoire of interests by exploring and teaching various activities.

Interference Current (IFC).   This modality may also be referred to as interferential electrical stimulation. See Physical agent modalities for further discussion.

Interferential Electrical Stimulation.   A physical agent modality that uses electrical current to treat pain and edema. See Physical agent modalities for further discussion and treatment.

Interpersonal Skills.   Verbal and nonverbal communication as a part of social skills. Knowing how to initiate a conversation, express support of another, showing humor, problem solve, and demonstrate self-control.

Intervention.   The application of treatments, techniques, methods, drugs, or surgery to improve the patient's condition.

Internal.   See Anatomical position.

Internal Rotation.   See Anatomical position.

Interphalangeal.   See Hand injuries.

Intrinsic Motivation.   The internal motivation to achieve or perform an activity without external rewards. For example, an artist will continue painting without expecting any reward or praise. Individuals with intrinsic motivation have an internal locus of control

Intrinsic Plus Grasp.   See Grasp.

Intrinsic-Plus Position.   A position recommended by James (1970) for immobilization of the injured hand. This position places the intrinsic muscles in an optimal position to help prevent atrophy. A hand that has atrophy of the intrinsic muscles will lose its ability to cup the palm/hand. This position places the MCP joints in flexion to near 90° degrees while allowing full extension of the PIP and DIP joints.

Inversion.   See Anatomical position.

Iontophoresis.   A physical agent modality that uses electrical current to drive ions, which are contained within topical medications, into underlying tissue for the purpose of promoting wound healing, or reducing pain, muscle spasm, calcium deposits, infection, scar tissue or edema. See Physical agent modalities for further discussion and treatment.

Isometric Contraction.   See Contraction.

Isotonic contraction.   See Contraction.

Job Burnout. A debilitating condition caused by chronic occupational stress, which results in depleted energy, lowered resistance to illness, job dissatisfaction, pessimism, increased inefficiency, and absenteeism.

Job Coach. A counselor or therapist who provides support to the employed client.

Joint Compression. A technique that can be used to either facilitate or inhibit Muscle tone. When heavy joint compression is applied, the joint receives more force than it regularly supports. For instance, through the act of pushing downward on the patient's shoulders, the therapist manually assists a patient who is prone on elbows. The patient is receiving more force through the shoulder joint than the shoulder usually supports when the patient is in this position. This technique facilitates Cocontraction of muscles around the joint. If light joint compression is applied, meaning the same or less force is applied than the joint is used to supporting, inhibition occurs. The main application of this type of compression occurs when a patient with hemiplegia lies supine and the therapist approximates the head of the humerus. See Motor Control Problems and Rood Approach for further discussion of facilitation and inhibition techniques.

Joint Mobilization. A technique in which the therapist to passively move a joint to its accessory motions prior to voluntary movement of that joint to achieve maximum ROM. Accessory motion, sometimes referred to as joint play, is nonvoluntary movement, which occurs at the joint as the bones glide over one another. If the bones are not gliding or rotating as they should, both passive and active ROM/movement will be hindered. Accessory motions include rotation, anterior-posterior glide, lateral glide, flexion and extension tilt, and distraction. A therapist must know the orthokinematics of the joint being

Joint Mobilization. *(continued)*

treated before attempting to restore joint play. Passive movement to promote each accessory motion at a joint should be completed for 30–60 seconds prior to ROM if the patient demonstrates impaired movement. Mobilization is appropriate for patients with limited ROM, pain from the joint capsule, meniscus displacement, tight ligaments, muscle guarding, or adhesions (Norkin & Levangie, 1992).

Contraindications/precautions

- Passive accessory motion should not be applied when a patient has hypermobility, infection, inflammation, effusion, osteoporosis, degenerative joint disease, unhealed fracture, or rheumatoid arthritis. Care should be taken if a patient has malignancy of the site being treated, excessive pain, or total joint replacement.

Techniques

- **Rhythmic Oscillations**: The bones are passively moved through either a small or large range of movement, at a rate of 2–3 oscillations per second. This type of mobilization may be used for patients who complain of pain.
- **Sustained Stretch or Distraction**: The bones are passively moved through the entire available range of movement and held in that position. Tiny oscillatory movements may be applied at the limit of range. This type of mobilization is used when accessory motion is tight and limits the patient's functional ROM.

Examples

- **Metacarpophalangeal Joint (MCP).** This joint is able to complete three motions: flexion/extension, abduction/adduction, and rotation. Before mobilization begins, the therapist must decide which way the moving bone glides at the articular surface. The head of the metacarpal is convex and the base of the proximal phalanx is concave; therefore, the base of the proximal phalanx moves on the metacarpal and glides in the same direction as the physiological motion being completed. Each MCP receives mobilization individually.

- *Distraction*. This is the first movement to be completed since the intraarticular space must be large enough to allow any ROM at the joint. The therapist should firmly hold the metacarpal bone with one hand, while using the other hand to grasp near the base of the proximal phalanx while the MCP is slightly flexed. The therapist gently pulls the phalanx distally to distract the joint.

- *Flexion/extension*. Again, the therapist firmly holds the metacarpal bone with one hand and the base of the proximal phalanx on the dorsal and volar surfaces with the other hand, while slightly flexing the MCP. The patient's hand is usually pronated during the procedure. The therapist gently pushes downward, while slightly distracting the joint, to produce a volar glide; then the therapist allows the bone to relax back to its original position. Volar glide helps increase flexion of the MCP. To increase extension at the MCP, dorsal glide is completed. The therapist begins mobilization with the same grasp as in the volar glide. The therapist gently pushes upward on the base of the proximal phalanx to produce a dorsal glide. The proximal phalanx is then allowed to relax back to its previous alignment.

- *Abduction/adduction*. The therapist holds the metacarpal bone and proximal phalanx with the same method used during flexion/extension, except the proximal phalanx should be held on the radial and ulnar surfaces. The therapist then slightly distracts the joint and gently pushes toward the radius, while the hand is pronated, to produce a radial glide. This glide helps increase ROM when completing abduction with the index and adduction with the ring and small digits. The joint should be allowed to relax back to its starting position. To help increase adduction with the index and abduction with the ring and small digits, the therapist should gently push the proximal phalanx toward the ulna. Again the joint is allowed to relax and return to its starting position.

Joint Mobilization

- *Rotation*. The therapist continues to hold the metacarpal bone and proximal phalanx in the above manner. The therapist then gently oscillates the base of the phalanx in a circle in one direction. The therapist should then complete circular motions with the phalanx moving in the opposite direction, since rotation can occur in either direction.

- **Wrist (radiocarpal) Joint**: This joint completes two motions: flexion/extension and radial/ulnar deviation. The proximal row of carpal bones are convex, so they move on the concave surface of the radius and radioulnar disk. As the carpal bones glide downward (toward the volar surface of the arm), the wrist is extended. During flexion at the wrist, the proximal carpal bones glide upward/dorsally. In this case, the accessory motion occurs in a direction opposite of the physiological movement.

  - *Distraction*: The therapist should palpate the wrist to grasp the proximal row of carpal bones with one hand, while holding the distal radius and ulna with the other hand. The therapist places the palms over the dorsal surface of the patient's wrist with the index fingers and thumbs as close together as possible while holding the proper structures. The therapist should stabilize the radius/ulna while gently pulling the hand outward from the wrist. The hand is then allowed to relax back to its previous position. This increases the intra-articular space, which will increase all ROM.

  - *Flexion/extension*: The therapist grasps the wrist using the same method that was used for distraction. The therapist slightly distracts the joint and gently pulls the proximal row of carpal bones upward (toward the dorsal surface of the arm) while the forearm is either pronated or in neutral. The hand relaxes back to its starting position. This dorsal glide helps increase wrist flexion. For extension, the proximal row of carpal bones are pushed in a volar direction to produce a volar glide, using the above positioning of the therapist and patient's hands.

- *Radial/ulnar deviation*: The therapist and patient begin in the same position as above; however, the therapist's palms are placed over the radial side of the wrist with the fingers wrapped around the ulnar side of the wrist. The therapist slightly distracts the joint and gently lifts the proximal row of carpal bones toward the radius. The hand should relax back to its starting position. Radial glide increases ulnar deviation. For radial deviation, the therapist pushes the proximal row of carpal bones toward the ulna to produce ulnar glide. The therapist always allows the joint to return to its original position unassisted.

Key Points of Control.   Specific areas of the body used by the therapist during Handling to help control movement patterns. The main key points used for controlling proximal movement include the shoulder, pelvis, and spine/ribcage. When controlling distal movement patterns, the hand and foot are key points. See Motor control problems and Neurodevelopmental treatment for further discussion of this type of treatment.

Kinesthesia.   A perceptual process or ability to understand and perceive the direction, amount, and position of movement in space. For example one's ability to throw a ball or use a hammer depends upon kinesthesia.

Klinefelter's Syndrome.   A male with this syndrome has three sex chromosomes, XXY. The person may develop primary male characteristics; however, he will most likely be infertile and develop few, if any, male secondary sex characteristics such as facial hair, etc. The person may also demonstrate learning disabilities in the areas of reading and verbal comprehension.

Kyphosis.   A concave curvature of the spine that may result from pathology or posterior pelvic tilt. See Pelvic tilt.

Labyrinthine righting. See <u>Reflexes and reactions</u>.

Lateral. See <u>Anatomical position</u>.

Laterality. Ability to use one side of the body, single hand or foot in purposeful activities such as eating with a fork, kicking a soccer ball, writing with a pencil, tossing a baseball, or using a screwdriver.

Lateral Prehension. This prehension pattern is comprised of opposition of the thumb to the radial side of the index finger (either the middle or distal phalanx). This pattern is used when turning a key or holding a fork.

Lateral Rotation. See <u>External rotation</u>.

Lead Pipe Rigidity. This type of rigidity is characterized by *constant* resistance to movement in any direction with no relaxation of the agonist or antagonist muscles occurring. This hypertonicity is uniform so that the same resistance is felt at any point in the affected joint's ROM. See <u>Rigidity</u> and <u>Cogwheel rigidity</u> for further discussion.

Learning. Cognitive ability to acquire new concepts and behaviors. Learning can occur through trial and error, such as in walking, riding a bicycle, and playing a musical instrument. Learning also involves memory as in learning how to read, rehearsing multiplication tables, and reciting a poem. Learning also involves imitation as in social skills and dancing. Learning can also include the formation of religious beliefs, values, ethical behavior, and occupational interests.

Learning Disability. A disorder affecting a person's ability to interpret visual and auditory stimuli and to integrate information processed by the brain. Difficulties result in spoken and written language, reading, calculating numbers, spelling, attending, and motor planning.

Learning Disability

Related Disabilities

- **Attention Deficit Hyperactivity Disorder (ADHD)**: symptoms of inattention, hyperactivity, and impulsiveness that interfere with an individual's ability to learn, work and engage in interpersonal and leisure activities.

- **Developmental Aphasia**: difficulty in understanding or expressing feelings and thoughts through speech, written language, or bodily gestures. It is caused by brain injury usually to the left hemisphere of brain (85% of time).

- **Dyonomia**: difficulty in remembering or retrieving names, words, a date, telephone numbers, passwords, or information during speaking or writing.

- **Dyscalculia**: difficulty in understanding and doing mathematics such as multiplication, division, fractions, and algebra.

- **Dysgraphia**: difficulty in writing letters legibly or written at an age-appropriate level.

- **Dyslexia**: difficulty in interpreting or reading written language. Difficulties in spelling, writing, and listening are associated with dyslexia.

- **Dyspraxia**: difficulty performing purposeful novel motor tasks in the proper sequence such as in dressing, driving a car, playing tennis, or brushing one's teeth.

- **Perceptual Disability**: dysfunction in discriminating, organizing, and processing visual, auditory, tactile, and kinesthetic information such as in reading or writing letters (b and d), differentiating in saying seer and sear, feeling metal or plastic, and throwing a ball.

- **Specific Learning Disability**: difficulty in processing that affects an area of learning, such as reading, writing, doing arithmetic, listening, or speaking; the disability is not caused by mental retardation, emotional disturbance, cultural differences, or sensory deficits such as blindness.

- **Sensory Integrative Dysfunction**: developmental disorder in which deficits in processing and integrating sensory input is hypothesized to result in problems in learning and behavior disorders in children.

- **Sensory Modulation Disorder**: individual over responds, under responds, or fluctuates in response to sensory input in a manner disproportional to that input (i.e., tactile defensiveness, gravitational insecurity).
  - *Tactile defensiveness*: defensive or fearful reaction to being touched or handled. The individual may complain or pull away from being touched and avoid activities that are messy and in engaging in body contact sports.
  - *Gravitational insecurity*: an emotional or fear reaction that is out of proportion to the actual danger of the vestibular-proprioceptive stimuli or position of the body in space (esp. when feet are off the ground).

Treatment Strategies and Materials

- **Accommodations**: computer software programs such as spell and grammar checks and allowing longer time to complete assignments.
- **Cognitive-behavioral techniques**
- **Role playing**
- **Behavioral rehearsal**
- **Relaxation therapy**
- **Stress management**
- **Assistive Technology**: equipment such as computers, audio and video recorders, and communication devices.
- **Environmental adaptation**: adjusting heights of tables and chairs, providing adapted equipment, and providing a learning environment free of distractions, all of which enable the individual to learn.
- **Metacognitive Teaching**: emphasizing the conscious learning of information through systematic practice, trial and error, rehearsal, and selection of the most effective ways to learn material such as through tape recorder or rewriting notes.
- **Multisensory Teaching**: incorporates multiple sensory channels such as auditory, visual, tactile, and kinesthetic in learning. For example, drawing a letter in sand while saying the letter.

Learning Disability

- **Resource Program**: classroom where the student has the opportunity for individual instruction and learning experiences outside the regular curriculum.
- **Sensory Integration Therapy**: techniques that involve the use of enhanced, controlled sensory stimulation in the context of a meaningful, self-directed activity to elicit an adaptive behavior.
- **Special Education Techniques**: specially designed instruction to fit the individual needs of a student with disabilities. Methods may include direct instruction in academic subjects and reading, writing, language, or arithmetic; adaptation of materials; or use of alternative methods. The interests of the student such as sports, fashion, popular music, automotive repair, or science fiction are incorporated into the learning exercises. The learning style of the student is considered such as active/passive, field independent/dependent, reflective/ impulsive, or verbal/auditory/tactile in structuring learning.

Leisure.　A major occupation and performance area that relates to the individual's use of free time. It is related to intrinsic motivation, quality of life, personal freedom, life satisfaction, relaxation, health, life style, amusement, self-actualization, and pleasure. Leisure occupation include a wide range of activities such as gardening, sports, hobbies, social clubs, music, and traveling, that are related to the specific interests of an individual. Cultural, psychological, social, developmental, family, and educational factors may influence leisure choices.

Level of Arousal.　A cognitive component that indicates an individual's alertness and responsiveness to environmental stimuli. An individual in a coma has little or no response when stimulated.

Limb Apraxia.　See Apraxia.

Limb Synergies.　A pattern of movement, involving various muscle contractions, which automatically occurs when one of the muscles (within the stereotypical movement) attempts to contract individually. These abnormal movement patterns are often present in persons who have hemiplegia. The upper and lower extremities can each demonstrate a Flexor and Extensor synergy. See Motor control problems and Movement therapy of Brunnstrom for treatment methods.

Locus of Control.   An individual's view that events can either be influenced by self (internal locus of control) or are predetermined or influenced by others (external locus of control).

Logical Positivism.   A philosophical approach to verifying reality. Logical positivists assert that reality is a result of sensory data.

Lordosis.   A convex curvature of the spine that may result from pathology or anterior pelvic tilt. See Pelvic tilt.

Low Back Pain (LBP).   One of the most common disabilities affecting millions of individuals in the industrial world It results in costs of millions of dollars in worker's compensation as well as creating severe problems in Self-care and performing Leisure activities.

Multifactorial Causes
- Structural impairments of the spinal column
- Prolonged static positions
- Incorrect continuous lifting
- Obesity
- Sedentary work
- Lack of exercise
- Stress also exacerbates the symptoms of LBP by creating tense and rigid muscles.

Symptoms
- A common finding in LBP is the presence of a herniated intervertebral disc that impacts on the spinal nerves. The pain may radiate in the lower extremities through the sciatic nerve.

143

Specific Treatments

- **Psychoeducational approach**: Teaching individuals to use
  - Proper lifting techniques (e.g., lifting objects from the floor by bending knees and keeping object close to the body in a squat position)
  - Preventative exercises in the morning including stretching the back muscles by bringing knees to axilla, tilting pelvis while in supine position and modified sit-ups. The exercises are individualized.
  - Ergonomics in performing Self-care activities, such as toileting, bed making, cooking, and laundering that reduce stress on the low back
  - Prescriptive exercises such as walking and bicycling that stretch back muscles while increasing muscle strength. Vary movements and plan short stretch breaks at work and at home.
  - Stress management techniques
- **Work Hardening**.
  - Simulating bending, lifting, carrying, standing and sitting positions.
  - Setting up graduated activities with goal of worker performing at 100% efficiency.
  - Using BTE or other functional evaluation to determine client's capacities.
- **Home Adaptation**.
  - Recommending alterations in client's home environment such as positioning of cabinets, and appliances, hand rails in bathroom and use of stools in raising legs while seated.
- **Expand Leisure Activities**.
  - Assisting the client to engage in occupations that are purposeful, meaningful and increase Muscle strength and Range of motion in back joints.
  - Consider gross motor activities, such as woodworking, pottery, bowling, swimming, gardening and bicy-

cling. See Coordination and Range of motion treatment methods.

Contraindications/Precautions

- Discontinue exercise if client experiences pain
- Observe for signs of depression in client that frequently accompany LBP
- Rule out malingering syndrome especially if client is receiving Worker's Compensation
- Monitor for muscle and joint substitutions in compensating for pain

Lower Motor Neuron Disorders. Lesions of the central nervous system may cause a loss of ventral horn cells or axons of the lower motor neurons, which are the cranial, spinal, or peripheral nerves, that innervate muscles. These are referred to as lower motor neuron lesions, and they result in decreased muscle tone or flaccidity, decreased Deep tendon reflexes or areflexia, and fasciculations (a twitching-like contraction of the muscle under the skin) of the muscle as well as atrophy. Disorders and diseases, which may result in a lower motor lesion, include poliomyelitis, postpolio syndrome, Guillain-Barré syndrome, radiculopathies, Myasthenia gravis, Amyotrophic lateral sclerosis, and botulism.

Macular Degeneration. A condition that results in degeneration of the macula of the retina which is the location of the highest concentration of rods and cones for vision. Degeneration begins at the macula and proceeds outwards; this may result in total blindness. See Blindness for further discussion of treatment.

Manual Contacts. Specific placement of the therapist's hands on the patient to help facilitate movement and provide sensory cues during treatment within the framework of PNF. The therapist should place his or her hands on the patient to help reinforce the desired movement; for example, if D_2 flexion is desired, then the therapist should place his or her hands on the patient's scapula to facilitate scapula elevation, rotation, and adduction. See Motor control problems, Proprioceptive neuromuscular facilitation for treatment and techniques.

Manual Muscle Test. A technique used to help the therapist identify the muscle strength of specific muscles and groups of muscles through maximal voluntary contraction (Hislop, Montgomery, & Connelly, 1995). The therapist usually tests a group of muscles together, which are responsible for the same action; these are called prime movers. Grades are then given for the *action* rather than for each individual muscle. During this test, the only tool used by the therapist is his or her hands. Because there is no objective measurement tool for this test, the same therapist should retest his or her patients to provide more reliability to the strength grades. This tool should not be used with a person who demonstrates spasticity, since the muscle contraction is not voluntary.

General Procedures
- The patient's joints should first be passively moved through their full available range of motion.
- The procedure should be explained to the patient followed by demonstration if needed.

Manual Muscle Test

- The patient should be allowed to rest for 2 minutes between tests if the same muscle is used to avoid inaccurate results from fatigue of the muscle.
- The patient should then be positioned so that movement is against gravity.
- The therapist should stabilize the stationary/proximal part of the joint without placing his or her hands over the contracting muscles, since stabilization helps isolate the proper movement and hinders substitutions.
- The patient is then asked to actively move the extremity through full ROM while the therapist palpates the muscle bellies or tendons of the prime movers to check that no substitution is occurring. If the patient actively moves through full ROM, the patient is asked to hold near the end position of range. After the patient is allowed to give maximal effort, the therapist resists the motion by pushing against the distal end of the moving bone toward the opposite motion. For example, if testing elbow flexion, the therapist pushes the forearm toward elbow extension. The therapist then grades the muscle strength.
- If the patient is unable to actively move the joint through its available ROM, the patient should be placed in a gravity-eliminated position. The patient is asked to complete AROM, and the muscle strength is graded by observing the motion the patient is able to accomplish. Maximum resistance should not be given if the patient requires a gravity-eliminated position to complete motion. This specific type of MMT is called the break test.
- The make test can also be used. In this type of test, the therapist provides resistance to the moving part of the joint as it moves through its range.

Muscle Grading Scales: The following numerical or letter-grading scales are explained together since the systems are both widely used by therapists.

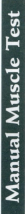

Manual Muscle Test

5	Normal	N	The part moves through full ROM against gravity and maximum resistance.
4	Good	G	The part moves through full ROM against gravity and moderate resistance.
3+	Fair plus	F+	The part moves through full ROM against gravity and minimal resistance.
3	Fair	F	The part moves through full ROM against gravity but with no resistance.
3−	Fair minus	F−	The part moves through partial (more than 50%) ROM against gravity.
2+	Poor plus	P+	The part moves through partial (less than 50%) ROM against gravity, or through full ROM in a gravity-eliminated position against minimal resistance.
2	Poor	P	The part moves through full ROM in gravity-eliminated position with no resistance.
2−	Poor minus	P−	The part moves through partial ROM in a gravity-eliminated position.
1	Trace	T	No motion is observed, but an increase in tone can be palpated.
0	Zero	0	No motion is observed and no tone can be palpated.

Functional Muscle Testing. This technique, which condenses the full MMT, may be completed in the interest of time rather than the full MMT. If this is the case, treatment should focus on strengthening groups of muscles, which complete actions, rather than individual muscles. This technique may also be used as a screening tool or if weakness is not the patient's primary symptom.

Procedure
- The patient sits upright in a chair or wheelchair.
- The therapist asks the patient to complete a specific motion, while the therapist stabilizes the joint to isolate movement and check for substitutions.
- If the patient is able to complete full AROM, the therapist applies resistance near the end of the range after asking the patient to hold the contraction.
- If the patient is not able to complete full AROM, the patient should be placed in a gravity-eliminated position, or the appropriate grade below 3 should be assigned to the motion.
- A therapist should use this form of muscle testing only after the therapist knows and understands the full MMT.

Contraindications/Precautions
- Muscle strength should not be measured in the presence of the following conditions: myositis ossificans, joint dislocation, surgery or repair to musculoskeletal structures at the site being tested, fractures which have not completely healed, inflammation, or pain.
- Precautions should be used if the patient has osteoporosis, a subluxation, joint laxity, hemophilia, abdominal surgery or hernia, a cardiovascular condition, takes muscle relaxants or pain medication, or has a condition which can be exacerbated by muscle fatigue.

Massage.   Manipulation, methodical pressure, friction, and kneading of the body to reduce stress, increase relaxation, and reduce muscle tension. Massage applied with firm pressure in a circular motion. This treatment method is often used over scars for Desensitization, as well as to help loosen scar tissue, which may be attaching to underlying structures and inhibiting movement.

Manual Muscle Test

Maximal Resistance. This term, when used within the framework of PNF, refers to the greatest amount of resistance which can be given during an <u>Isometric contraction</u> without breaking the contraction, or during an <u>Isotonic contraction</u> without disrupting the movement of the body part. It *does not* refer to the greatest amount of resistance that the therapist can apply during movement. See <u>Motor control problems</u>, <u>Proprioceptive neuromuscular facilitation</u> for further techniques.

MCP. Metacarpophalangeal.

Medial. See <u>Anatomical position</u>.

Medial Rotation. See <u>Anatomical position</u>.

Median Plane. See <u>Anatomical position</u>.

Medicaid. Federally mandated entitlement program that provides medical care for individuals who are indigent.

Medical Model. The traditional approach to diagnosing, preventing, and treating diseases. It is based on the scientific method of hypothesis testing, and experimental design. In the medical model the physician focuses on detecting disease and treating it primarily through drugs and surgery. The physician is seen as the expert in treating the patient. A client-centered approach, behavioral medicine, or alternative medicine, and holistic medicine are contrasted with the traditional medical model, which has been attacked as being reductionistic.

Medicare. Federally mandated entitlement program that reimburses hospitals, physicians, and health care workers in providing services to individuals 65 years and older.

Meditation. Relaxation activity where the individual takes a comfortable position in a quiet environment, regulating breathing, and having a physically relaxed and mentally calm attitude while focusing on a mental image or word.

Memory. Cognitive ability to retrieve or recall information after brief, short-term or long periods of time. Memory is a component of information processing that involves learning information, storing it, and then recalling it. Memory deficits such as in brief or short-term recall are major symptoms in individuals with Alzheimer's disease. Therapists can use purposeful activities such as with cards or puzzles to stimulate memory. See Cognitive-perceptual deficits for further discussion and treatment.

Ménière's Disease. A condition which results in vertigo, nausea, vomiting, and may lead to total deafness.

Mental Retardation (MR). Developmental disability characterized by subnormal intellectual aptitude potential with an IQ below 70, and significant limitations in adaptive behavior skills in at least two of the following areas : communication, Self-care, home and community living, Social skills, health and safety, Leisure activities, Work and functional academics. MR can range from mild, moderate, or severe to profound disability.

> *Causes.* There are many causes of mental retardation that ranges from genetic, prenatal, paranatal and postnatal developmental, addiction to drugs and alcohol in the mother and sociocultural factors such as poverty and deprivation.

> *Prevention.* Preventing mental retardation include dietary treatment of children with phenylketonuria (PKU), thyroid replacement therapy for children with hypothyroidism, folic acid as a dietary supplement for mother, blood exchanges for children born with erthythroblastosis and Rh factor, the use of vaccines to prevent rubella during pregnancy and Psychoeducational programs to teach mothers at risk good prenatal care. Other interventions in the environment include the use of seat belts, bicycle helmets, and the removal of lead from old buildings. In general good prenatal and

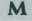
Mental Retradation

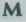

pediatric care can prevent many instances of mental retardation.

Prevalence. Approximately 7 million individuals or 3% of the general population in the United States have mental retardation. Of this population about 87% will be mildly or moderately affected with mental retardation with IQs above 50. Thirteen percent of individuals with mental retardation will have severe or profound cognitive deficits.

Treatment (See Down syndrome) The treatment of individuals with MR is based on a holistic approach taking into consideration the individual's potential and needs. The therapist should consider:

- Self-care activities and provide a home program with parent's cooperation
- Leisure activities that are meaningful to client, age appropriate and provide sensory and motor stimulation
- Work activities such as supportive employment with a job coach, sheltered work or supervised volunteer experiences
- Assistive technology devices that help the individual to learn, communicate, ambulate, increase self-care skills, work, and engage in leisure sports and recreation

Metabolic Equivalent Levels (MET). A measure of the oxygen used by a person's body while completing activities and maintaining the body's metabolic processes such as respiration, body temperature, etc. The energy required by a person who is resting in a semi-reclined chair is equal to 1 MET.

Equivalencies
- 1.5–2 MET = Standing, driving, typing, or walking at 1 m.p.h.
- 2–3 MET = Playing piano, level bicycling, or walking at 2 m.p.h.
- 3–4 MET = Pushing a light mower, golf with a pull cart, or walking at 3 m.p.h.

Metabolic Equivalent Levels (MET)

- 4–5 MET = Raking leaves, hoeing, ballroom dancing, or walking at 3.5 m.p.h.
- 5–6 MET = Skating, canoeing, or walking at 4 m.p.h.
- 6–7 MET = Water skiing, light downhill skiing, singles tennis, snow shoveling, or walking at 5 m.p.h.
- 7–8 MET = Vigorous downhill skiing, basketball, ice hockey, or jogging
- 8–9 MET = Fencing, vigorous basketball, or running
- 10+ MET = Handball or running
- Most Self-care activities require under 3 MET with the exclusion of bathing/showering, washing hair, and toileting

Principles of Energy Conservation

- Plan ahead to use the most direct or easiest method for completion and reduce wasted motion.
- Sit while working, when possible.
- Avoid unnecessary tasks.
- To eliminate trips during a task, gather all the necessary tools prior to starting.
- Items that are used often should be lightweight and kept within easy reach.
- Combine tasks when possible. For example, take one trip to the kitchen and complete all tasks there to reduce the number of trips between rooms.
- Use power tools, such as an electric can opener or mixer, to do the work when possible.
- Allow gravity to assist work rather than oppose it.
- Schedule rest breaks before becoming fatigued.
- Avoid stressful positions or situations such as the following: a hot, humid environment or quick temperature changes; reaching above the head; bending at the waist to reach to the floor or lower extremities; standing for prolonged periods of time; isometric contractions, such as pulling or pushing, which can cause a person to hold one's breath; exertion following meals since the distended stomach places pressure against the diaphragm; excessive bilateral extremity use; and overexertion.

Metabolic Equivalent Levels (MET)

Examples

- Spread tasks out over the day or week. Alternate between heavy and light tasks.
- Complete tasks often to keep the amount of work small. If dishes are left until the end of the week, a large amount of energy will be needed for the task. Doing a few dishes each day requires only a little energy.
- Organize trips to eliminate backtracking.
- Delegate tasks to family members or friends when possible.
- Soak dirty dishes before washing them, and then allow them to air-dry.
- Use fitted sheets.
- Schedule essential tasks, which require more energy during peak hours of the day when the person has the most energy.
- Divide lengthy tasks into smaller tasks. For example, iron for a short period of time and different intervals during the day or week.
- Schedule frequent rest breaks, which last 10–15 minutes, especially following a heavy task.
- Do not start tasks, such as carrying a heavy item for a long distance, which do not allow a person to stop and rest.
- Avoid rushing.
- Avoid unnecessary stairs, bending, reaching, stretching, carrying, lifting, and holding.
- Use a utility cart on wheels for transporting items.
- Use the foot to close a low cabinet door rather than bending over.
- Slide a pan along the countertop from the sink to the stove.
- Use assistive technology to make tasks easier. A nonskid mat will help stabilize pans or dishes. Long-handled reachers or dressing sticks will help a person don socks or pants.
- Maintain normal body weight.

- Use good body mechanics during activities. Good posture can help prevent fatigue. Wear comfortable, supportive shoes, which will assist with proper posture.
- Remember that emotions expend energy also.

See Work simplification for more techniques to make activities easier and more manageable.

Microcurrent Electrical Neuromuscular Stimulation (MENS). A physical agent modality that uses electrical current to help reduce acute or chronic pain, reduce inflammation, reduce spasm, and promote healing of bones, nerves, or connective tissue. The efficacy of this modality is controversial. See Physical agent modalities for further discussion and treatment.

MMT. See Manual muscle test.

Mobile Arm Support. An assistive device to assist a patient who has weakness or decreased ROM with feeding or other functional activities. This device may also be referred to as a balanced forearm orthosis. It attaches to the frame of the wheelchair along the edge of the seat back to assist the patient with activities. Persons with the following diagnoses may benefit from this device: spinal cord injury, Guillain-Barré syndrome, muscular dystrophy, amyotrophic lateral sclerosis, and poliomyelitis. To benefit from the device and increase function, a patient should have muscle strength at the elbow and shoulder which has been assessed with a Manual muscle test at a level 1–3. See Assistive devices for further discussion of adaptive equipment.

Model of Human Occupation (MOHO). Occupational therapy frame of reference that is based on the theory of general systems. Role acquisition, environmental and temporal adaptation, and skill development are emphasized in treatment. Volition, habituation, and performance are key concepts (Kielhofner, 1997).

Modeling Behavior.   A technique used in behavior therapy to help the client acquire social skills by observing and then imitating behavior

Mood Disorders.   Disturbances of affect such as <u>Depression</u>, mania, and <u>Bipolar disorders</u>.

Moral Treatment.   A movement during the 19th century that developed as a reaction to the inhumane care of the mentally ill who up until that time were abused and poorly treated. Arts and crafts, farming, and creative activities were emphasized in moral treatment.

Moro Reflex.   See <u>Reflexes and reactions</u>.

Motor Control.   The ability to use the body in purposeful and versatile activities such as in learning how to dance, riding a bicycle, engaging in a sport, or doing intricate hand work in knitting or crocheting.

Motor Control Problems

Traditional Approaches to Treatment. The following theories of rehabilitation underlie treatment for persons not able to control voluntary movement. These approaches share the following common assumptions: sensation is an important precursor to producing voluntary movement, motor control reoccurs in a developmental sequence like that which occurs when a child grows, and the central nervous system is able to be reorganized. Contemporary theories on motor control question these assumptions and dispute some of the following techniques. Very few, if any, studies have been completed recently to check the validity of these approaches; however, some of the techniques and ideas supported in the past may still benefit patients with movement difficulties.

Rood approach. The basic assumption is that sensation is able to produce motor responses.

General principles
- Muscle tone can be normalized and motor responses can be evoked with appropriate sensory stimuli.
- Treatment occurs sequentially from the patient's current developmental level to higher levels of motor control.
- Purposeful activity or movement automatically programs the nervous system to facilitate the correct muscles involved in an activity; therefore, the patient can focus on a functional goal rather than a movement.
- Motor learning occurs through repetition of a movement.

Treatment
- Sensory input
  - Facilitation
    - → Fast Brushing over the skin of a muscle with a soft brush (avoid the face, head, and ear).
    - → Light moving touch or Stroking with a fingertip, soft brush or cotton swab (suggested frequency is 3–5 strokes with 30 seconds between).
    - → Icing (suggested frequency is 3 quick strokes). Avoid icing the face, neck, ear, and midline of the body. Icing the midline of the body of a patient with a C4–C5 spinal cord injury can elicit Autonomic dysreflexia and cause seizures. Also avoid icing with patients who have cardiac problems as icing the region of the left shoulder can cause angina.
    - → Heavy Joint compression can facilitate Cocontraction at a joint.
    - → Quick Stretch, such as, quickly bending the elbow to stretch the triceps.

→ Intrinsic stretch, usually through pressure applied by a cone or handle, which can promote Cocontraction at the shoulder.

→ Stretch pressure (which should last a suggested duration of 3 seconds) by placing firm pressure while pulling both hands apart while stretching a superficial muscle with the fingertips of both thumbs and first two digits.

→ Resistance used in an isotonic manner so that the muscle contracts in a shortened length.

→ Tapping to a muscle or its tendon before or during a contraction (suggested frequency is 3–5 taps).

→ Vestibular stimulation mainly in the form of fast rocking. Slow, rhythmic rocking can have the opposite effect of inhibition.

→ Inversion, mainly to facilitate neck, trunk, and selected limb muscles.

→ Vibration applied with light pressure over a muscle belly, parallel with the muscle fibers (suggested duration is not more than 2 minutes).

→ Osteopressure over a bony prominence; however this should be preceded by light moving touch.

• Inhibition
    → Neutral warmth, such as wrapping the patient's body in a blanket for 5–10 minutes, may decrease muscle tone.

    → Gentle rocking while applying traction and/or compression to the joint being moved, as in the case with the patient's head, shoulder girdle, pelvis, or lower extremities.

    → Slow Stroking along both sides of the spinous processes of the patient's vertebrae, beginning at the occiput and continuing to the coccyx and alternating hands so that as the left hand reaches the coccyx, the right hand is beginning at the occiput.

→ Slow "log" Rolling of a patient from a side-lying position into prone position and back into sidelying so that the patient's shoulders and hips roll simultaneously; some segmental rolling can be completed as well to separate the hips from the trunk so that the patient is able to turn his or her trunk independently from turning his or her hips.

→ Light Joint compression less than body weight usually applied through two joints (e.g., approximating the head of the humerus into the glenohumeral joint by holding onto the proximal forearm while the patient's elbow is comfortably flexed and the humerus is slightly abducted). Once the tone begins to decrease, small circular movements can reduce pain in the shoulder and allow for greater ROM (this can also be completed through the elbow and wrist with the elbow flexed comfortably and the wrist held in extension).

• Deep Pressure to the tendinous insertion of a muscle.

• Maintained Stretch of a muscle for 1–2 minutes at its greatest length to lessen the effect of tone on a muscle during movement.

Levels of Motor Control. Treatment should proceed in this developmental order:

• Shortening and lengthening of muscles to produce Mobility at a distal joint (e.g., a baby shaking a rattle)

• Cocontraction of muscles around a proximal joint to

produce Stability (e.g., a baby learning to sit up)
- Mobility of proximal segments upon the Stability of distal segments (e.g. a baby rocking back and forth in quadruped)
- Skilled and controlled Mobility of distal segments on Stability of proximal segments (e.g., walking or reaching)

Eight Functional Motor Patterns. This theory believes that a patient will develop the above levels of motor control as he or she is progressed through the following sequence of patterns:

- *Supine withdrawal*: The patient lies on his or her back with back flexed, hips flexed and abducted, shoulders adducted and elbows flexed with extended hands toward his or her face.
- *Roll over*: The patient's upper and lower extremity flex as the patient rolls toward the opposite side (e.g. the right arm and leg flex as the patient rolls to the left).
- *Pivot prone*: The patient lies in prone with the shoulders abducted, extended, and externally rotated; lower extremities extended; and neck and head extended so that only the area of the patient's trunk around T10 level is touching the ground.
- *Neck cocontraction*: The patient lies in prone and is able to extend his neck and head against gravity.
- *Prone on elbows*: The patient again lies in prone with the neck/head extended and is able to flex the elbows and place weight on the elbows/forearms.
- *All fours (quadruped)*: The patient bears weight on both knees and hands with the elbows extended, shoulder flexed, hips flexed and neck/head extended.
- *Standing:* The patient bears weight on both feet with upper and lower extremities extended.
- *Walking*: The patient is able to stand, push off the floor with one foot, swing through with that same foot, strike the floor with that same heel, and repeat the process with the other foot.

Movement Therapy of Brunnstrom. (Brunnstrom, 1970, 1996). This theory is particularly concerned with the rehabilitation of patients who have suffered a stroke.

Assumptions

- Normal development involves the reorganization of spinal cord and brainstem Reflexes and reactions into purposeful movement; therefore, reflexes can assist the recovery of normal movement following stroke.
- Sensory stimuli can elicit motion.
- The recovery of movement progresses from synergies, which are movement patterns, which involve the entire involved limb, to normal voluntary movements.
- Learning through practice of the new voluntary movements, most effectively done through the incorporation of the movements into daily or purposeful activities, must be completed.

General Principles

- Treatment should progress according to normal motor development: reflexes to voluntary to functional movement.
- Reflexes, associated reactions, proprioceptive facilitation, and/or exteroceptive facilitation should be used to elicit movement when no motion is present.
- When the patient begins to demonstrate voluntary movement, he or she should be asked to complete an Isometric contraction (holding). After the patient has demonstrated success with this, an Eccentric contraction (lengthening) should be performed, with a Concentric contraction (shortening) being the final learned movement.
- Reversal of movement should also be stressed each treatment, for example, after practicing

161

Motor Control Problems

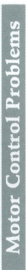

flexion, the patient should also be asked to complete extension.

- Facilitation methods such as reflexes or exteroceptive stimuli should be removed from treatment as soon as the patient demonstrates voluntary control of movement.
- The patient's decision for voluntary movement is stressed to help overcome the patterns of movement or synergies so that the patient is able to move one part of the extremity without the others automatically responding.
- Practice, practice, practice while including functional activities to decrease the synergistic patterns and increase the patient's purposeful movement.

Terms Used in Movement Therapy

- Associated reactions: abnormal movement, usually in the form of a synergy, which occurs in the affected extremity when the patient attempts a resisted or rapid movement with the unaffected extremity. For example, when resisting flexion with the unaffected arm, the affected arm will demonstrate involuntary flexion; and likewise, resisted extension in the unaffected arm will produce extension with the affected arm. In the lower extremities, the results are reversed so that resisted flexion in the unaffected leg produces extension in the affected leg. Ramiste's phenomenon is a term used for a specific associated reaction when resistance against hip abduction or adduction in the noninvolved lower extremity elicits the same motion in the involved extremity.
- Homolateral limb synkinesis: the associated reaction that occurs between extremities on the same side of the body. For example,

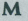

when the patient attempts to flex the affected arm, involuntary flexion in the leg may be elicited.

- <u>Specialized associated reactions</u>: occur in the hand of someone with hemiplegia include:
  - <u>Proximal traction response</u>: stretch to any of the flexor muscles of the affected extremity results in a flexor synergy, or flexion of all the flexor muscles in that extremity
  - <u>Grasp reflex</u>: results in flexion and adduction of the fingers when deep pressure is applied to the affected palm and moved distally toward the fingers, especially on the radial side of the hand.
  - <u>Instinctive grasp reaction</u>: elicited by placing an object in the patient's affected hand and results in the hand grasping the item with an inability to release the object.
  - <u>Instinctive avoiding reaction</u>: results in the hyperextension of the thumb and fingers of the affected hand when the affected arm is moved forward and upward.
  - <u>Souques finger phenomenon</u>: the action of the affected fingers involuntarily extending when the affected shoulder is flexed.
- <u>Limb synergies</u>: stereotyped patterns of movement which begin as involuntary reactions which produce abnormal movement that is not under the patient's control, but which can hopefully be modified to help produce voluntary, controlled and normal movement.
  - <u>Flexor synergy</u>: In the upper extremity, the pattern includes elbow flexion (the strongest motion of the synergy), scapular

retraction and/or elevation, forearm supination, and shoulder abduction and external rotation (the two weakest parts of the synergy). The motions of the hand and wrist may vary from one patient to another. In the lower extremity, the components include hip flexion, abduction, and external rotation; knee flexion; dorsiflexion and inversion of the ankle; and dorsiflexion of the toes. Functional activities, which use this synergy, include carrying items such as a purse or briefcase, putting on eyeglasses, or feeding oneself. Bilateral pushing and pulling, such as sanding or polishing, alternately use both the flexor and extensor synergies.

- Extensor synergy: In the upper extremity, the components include shoulder horizontal adduction and internal rotation (the strongest two motions of the synergy), scapular protraction, elbow extension, and forearm pronation. Again, hand and wrist motions vary; however, a commonly demonstrated pattern is wrist extension with finger flexion. In the lower extremity, the pattern includes hip extension, adduction, and internal rotation; knee extension; plantar flexion and inversion of the ankle; and plantar flexion of the toes. Functional activities that use this synergy include holding an object with the affected extremity while working on it with the nonaffected extremity, placing the affected arm through a sleeve of a shirt or coat, or wiping off a table or countertop.

- Typical upper extremity posturing: Seen in

the patient with hemiplegia; may result from spasticity with both synergies developing simultaneously in the affected arm. Subsequently, the strongest components of each synergy are manifested in shoulder adduction and internal rotation, elbow flexion, forearm pronation, and then most generally, wrist and finger flexion.

- Stages of recovery in the arm of a patient who has experienced a stroke.
  - Flaccidity: No voluntary movement noted.
  - Spasticity: starting to develop, and synergies developing with flexion usually developing prior to extension.
  - Increased spasticity but some voluntary movement beginning during synergies.
  - Spasticity is decreasing and some voluntary movement apart from synergy, usually (a) hand behind body, (b) arm to forward-horizontal position, and (c) pronation-supination with elbow flexed to 90°.
  - Spasticity continues decreasing and more movement occurs which is independent from synergies, usually (a) arm to side-horizontal position, (b) arm forward and overhead, and (c) pronation-supination with elbow fully extended.
  - Spasticity is minimal and joint movements are completed with nearly normal movement patterns.
- Stages of recovery in the hand of a patient who has experienced a stroke.
  - Flaccidity: No voluntary movement noted.
  - Slight finger flexion possible.
  - Hook or mass grasp with no voluntary release.

- Slight finger extension and lateral prehension with release completed by thumb movement.
- <u>Palmar prehension</u>, <u>gross cylindrical</u> or <u>spherical grasp</u>, and increased finger extension with the fingers acting together as a unit.
- Full and voluntary finger extension and separate voluntary finger movements with increased ability to complete all prehension patterns.

Rehabilitation of Trunk Control. The patient is pushed in a direction so that trunk muscle contraction is facilitated to help restore the patient to an upright position. The patient should be encouraged to return to the upright position actively; however, the patient will most likely need assistance with this until the muscles have strengthened. Also, the patient should be guarded when he or she is pushed off balance to protect the patient from being hurt if he or she responds poorly to these activities at first.

1. The first step is facilitating contraction of the trunk muscles on the noninvolved side by gently pushing the patient toward the involved side. Once the person has acquired this skill, the therapist proceeds to step 2.
2. Next, the muscles on the involved side are facilitated by pushing the patient toward the noninvolved side.
3. Trunk flexion is practiced while the patient supports the involved arm with the noninvolved arm while sitting. The patient is assisted with forward flexion by the therapist. As the patient slowly bends forward, the therapist helps support the patient's upper extremities so that some shoulder flexion occurs while the patient is focusing on trunk control. The patient actively extends back to the upright position.
4. Trunk extension is practiced with the patient sitting in a

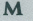

chair without a back support. The patient is assisted with backward extension while supporting the involved arm as described above, and encouraged to actively flex back to the upright position.

5. Trunk rotation is the final motion that is facilitated. Again, the involved arm is supported in the above manner while the therapist assists the patient in rotating his or her arm and trunk in one direction while rotating the patient's head in the opposite direction. This method uses the Tonic neck and Tonic lumbar reflexes as a means of beginning the shoulder movements of the upper extremity synergies.

Rehabilitation of Upper Extremity Control. As the upper extremity recovers, the hand may return at a different rate of recovery than the shoulder; therefore the stages and steps of regaining control are divided into proximal upper extremity and wrist/hand.

1. **Proximal Upper Extremity Control**. Treatment proceeds according to the stage of recovery of the patient's upper extremity.

   a. During stages 1 and 2 when the patient's arm is mostly flaccid, the goal is to elicit muscle tone and limb synergies through the use of reflexes and associated reactions. The flexor synergy, usually the first to develop, may be produced through resistance to the noninvolved upper extremity during shoulder elevation or elbow flexion. Tapping the upper and middle trapezius, rhomboids, and biceps can facilitate it. Elbow flexion, which is the strongest component of the flexion synergy, usually develops first.

   b. The next goal is to have the patient begin to develop voluntary control of the synergy. Upper extremity control begins with scapular elevation. The therapist places the patient's involved arm on a table so that the shoulder is abducted and the elbow is flexed. Next, the therapist places his or her hands on the patient's upper trapezius area and on the lateral side of the head to provide resistance as the patient is asked to hold the head still and resist having the head laterally flexed toward the noninvolved side. This motion is the beginning of lateral neck flexion toward the involved side, which may help initiate scapular elevation since the upper trapezius performs both motions. When contraction begins in the trapezius on the involved side, the patient continues to work against the therapist's resistance while concentrating on attempting to laterally flex the head to the involved side and elevating the affected shoulder. As the contraction strengthens and motion is detected, the therapist should use an associated reaction to help produce movement by placing a hand on the noninvolved shoulder/scapula and asking the patient to elevate the noninvolved shoulder. If an associated reaction occurs, the involved shoulder will also elevate during this activity. The next step is to provide resistance against shoulder/scapula elevation on the involved side as well as on the noninvolved side while the patient is asked to hold the contraction. Individual elevation of the involved scapula is practiced next while using facilitory techniques such as tapping or stroking if needed. The therapist helps the patient elevate the scapula and is then told to hold the contraction. The patient practices eccentric contraction of the shoulder when releasing the contraction slowly and lowering the shoulder back into place. Next, a Concentric contraction is attempted by asking the patient to raise the involved shoulder toward his or her ear. Care should be taken to assist the patient with the remainder of the upper extremity as Subluxation may have occurred and can cause the patient pain during the activity. The head of the humerus should be approximated and the arm abducted so that proper Scapulohumeral rhythm can

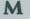
occur. The next motions to practice, which are the other components of the flexor synergy, are shoulder abduction, external rotation, and forearm supination.

c. Reversal of the flexor synergy movements, which are usually completed from the beginning of the above protocol, help develop voluntary control of the extensor synergy. Again, associated reactions may help the involved arm complete the correct contraction. The extensor synergy may be produced through resistance to the noninvolved upper extremity during horizontal adduction. Horizontal adduction is facilitated by resisting the noninvolved arm while holding the involved arm midway between horizontal adduction and abduction and asking the patient to bring his or her arms together. Elbow extension is elicited through a technique named Rowing. The therapist sits facing the patient with her arms crossed at the wrists and grasps the patient's hands, so that the therapist's right hand is holding the patient's right hand and left hand is to left hand. The patient sits with his or her arms supinated and flexed at the elbows. The therapist places his or her hands in the patient's palms so that the therapist is in pronation. The patient is asked to actively extend the noninvolved elbow while the therapist assists the involved arm extend. As the patient extends, the patient's hands are guided so that the patient begins to pronate and cross the arms toward the opposite knees while the therapist supinates and uncrosses his or her arms. Once a contraction is felt in the involved arm, the therapist asks the patient to hold the contraction in near full extension while the therapist provides resistance. The therapist guides the patient's arms back into an uncrossed, supinated, and flexed elbow position while the therapist again pronates and crosses her arms. Again, the therapist resists elbow extension in the noninvolved upper extremity to help evoke an associated reaction in the involved arm. Resistance is then given against the involved extremity's action once a contraction has been produced in the affected arm. Once the extensor synergy has developed, voluntary movement is reinforced through resistance against near full elbow extension. When active control of the extensor synergy is noted, bilateral Weight bearing on extended arms may begin. One method for weight bearing is to have the patient place his or her arms on a low stool in front of him or her while seated and support weight on both arms. Extension may be facilitated through stroking or Tapping the affected arm's triceps during the activity. The patient then progresses to unilateral weight bearing on the involved extremity only. Any activity in which the patient supports an object with the involved extremity while working on it with the noninvolved extremity can fulfill this requirement. Once the involved triceps produces active extension, resistance is given while completing the motion. Further facilitation methods include the use of reflexes such as the Assymetrical tonic neck reflex (watching the involved extremity during motion), the Tonic labyrinthine reflex (placing the patient in supine), or having the patient work on extension with the forearm in pronation which facilitates the extensor synergy.

d. Next, the extremity is facilitated to produce movement apart from the synergy. This begins by breaking up the motions that combine to form a synergy. For example, in the extensor synergy, the patient is encouraged to extend the involved elbow while the therapist guides the patient's extremity into shoulder abduction or supination, which challenges the synergy's pattern of shoulder adduction and pronation.

e. Voluntary movement is encouraged which combines aspects of both synergies in increasingly complex variations so that the effect of the synergies on movement decreases and willed movement increases. During this stage of rehabilitation, the therapist no longer uses associated reactions or reflexes to produce movement. Instead, the therapist isolates movement so that muscle groups can begin working independently of one another. Three specific movements deviating from synergy are listed below.

- Hand behind body may be easier for the patient to complete while standing if the patient demonstrates good balance. The patient combines shoulder abduction with elbow extension and forearm pronation in order to stroke the dorsal surface of the hand against the patient's back. This part of the activity provides sensory input and gives the voluntary movement a goal or direction. A swinging motion of the arm combined with trunk rotation can help assist the patient in getting the arm behind the back, or the therapist can actively assist the motion so that the patient completes the activity of stroking the back. The action should be practiced so that the therapist needs less help until the patient can complete the activity independently. Functional activities, which use this motion, include donning a belt or tucking a shirttail into pants.

- Shoulder flexion to a forward-horizontal position while extending the elbow is the second motion deviating from synergy. Again, the therapist may passively assist the patient if he or she is unable to complete the activity; however, facilitation should be used for the movements. Then "Place and hold" activities can be completed with active motion being the final goal. Functional activities, which use this motion, include any vertically mounted game or sponge painting.

- Pronation and supination while flexing the elbow to 90° is the final motion during stage 4 of upper extremity recovery .Supination should not be a problem since it is normally combined with elbow flexion in the flexor synergy. The therapist can begin by resisting pronation while the elbow is extended, and the therapist can then gradually bring the elbow into flexion while practicing pronation. Functional activities, which use this motion, include opening a door with a doorknob, using a screwdriver, or turning dials.

f. Movement in stage 5 of recovery involves increasingly complex movement, which is getting farther away from synergy but does not require excess force. Again, three specific movements are noted below.

- Arm raised to side-horizontal is the first movement to prove disassociation of the synergies. This motion combines full shoulder abduction with elbow extension. Proof that the synergies are still influencing movement include elbow flexion while abduction occurs or a drifting of the extremity toward horizontal adduction while the elbow is extended. The motion should be practiced until the patient can successfully demonstrate this motion. Functional activities, which use this motion, include placing objects on a strategically placed table, table tennis, and driving golf balls.

- Arm forward and overhead requires upward scapular rotation, so passive mobilization should be completed if the patient has spastic retractors or a weak serratus anterior. Retraining of the serratus anterior involves the patient placing the extremity in shoulder flexion and horizontal adduction and then trying to reach forward. Facilitation can be given through quick stretches into scapular retraction and then asking the patient to hold the scapula in that position. Next, the patient is asked to hold while the serratus is contracted and the scapula is protracted. As the serratus increases in strength, the shoulder is flexed in increasing increments until the arm is in the overhead position.

Functional activities, which use this motion, include sanding on an incline, shooting baskets, or painting a wall.

- Supination and pronation with the elbow extended is the final motion during this stage of recovery. Brunnstrom (1970, 1996) gave no special treatment recommendations to help disassociate supination from elbow extension. One activity, which could be used, is performing ball-handling skills. The patient would grasp a ball with both hands and arms out-stretched while rotating it so that first the affected arm was on top of the ball (pronating) and the unaffected arm was under the ball (supinating), and then the ball could be rotated so that the arms did the opposite motion of pronation/supination.

g. The final stage of recovery is willed movement; however, many patients with hemiplegia do not reach this stage.

2. **Rehabilitation of the Hand and Wrist**

a. Rehabilitation begins during Stage 1 when the patient's hand is flaccid. If the patient can initiate no finger flexion, then the therapist should give a quick stretch to the scapula adductors on the patient's affected side, which causes the fingers to slightly flex due to a traction response.

b. Once Grasp begins, the patient's wrist has a tendency to flex also. Treatment should focus on stabilizing the wrist during finger movement. This should first be attempted with the elbow in full extension, which helps facilitate wrist extension, and with the therapist supporting the patient's wrist. The therapist asks the patient to squeeze or strongly flex the fingers while the therapist facilitates contraction of the wrist extensor muscles. Once a contraction is felt in the wrist extensors, the therapist should discontinue support of the wrist during the "squeezing" or finger flexing and ask the patient to hold the contraction. Again, wrist extension can be facilitated, if necessary, through tapping. When the patient is able to grasp without flexing the wrist during full elbow extension, practice should occur while the elbow is slowly moved into a flexed position.

c. Next, finger flexion is inhibited and extension is facilitated through various techniques. One technique is placing the thumb in abduction/extension and then slowly pronating and supinating the patient's forearm, but especially emphasizing supination and holding the thumb more firmly during supination. Stroking or Tapping can be done on the dorsal surface of the wrist and hand to help the flexion relax. Light tapping can also be done to the dorsal surfaces to the patient's fingers while holding the patient's forearm in supination, so that the fingers slightly flex toward the palm, which gives a quick stretch to the extensors of the fingers. Following relaxation of the flexion, the patient's arm should be pronated and raised above horizontal (Souque's phenomenon) to assist with extension. Care should be taken to avoid maximum effort, as this can again increase flexor tension. Once the patient is able to extend the hand above head, practice should occur as the arm is slowly lowered. Any functional grasp and release activity can help the patient practice extension.

d. Lateral prehension release is practiced next. The therapist can help facilitate the patient's lifting the thumb from the side of the index finger by stroking over the abductor pollicis longus tendon. Once the patient is able to release lateral prehension, then the patient is encouraged to practice using and holding lateral prehension. Functional activities to practice this motion include using a key or holding and then releasing a book.

e. After the patient is able to extend the fingers and successfully release objects, more complex prehensile patterns can be practiced such as <u>Palmar prehension</u>, <u>Spherical grasp</u>, or <u>Cylindrical grasp</u>.

f. The final stage is individual finger movements. Functional activities such as typing, using an adding machine, or playing piano can be used; however the patient should be warned that he or she may not recover completely.

Proprioceptive Neuromuscular Facilitation (PNF) Approach. This approach is based on overall muscle movement patterns rather than individual muscle contractions. It can be used to treat patients with various conditions such as <u>Parkinson's disease</u>, spinal cord injury, arthritis, stroke, head injury, and <u>Hand injuries</u>.

General Principles.

• All persons have potential that has not been fully developed (Voss, 1967). Therefore, all persons have the ability to make progress and further develop from their current state. This philosophy also pertains to therapy, so that a patient can use a strong or able part to help a weaker part become further developed. For example, a patient with a flaccid upper extremity can use his or her strong upper extremity to help increase movement in the affected arm.

• Normal development proceeds in a cervicocaudal and proximodistal direction (Voss, 1967). Treatment should adhere to this model, so that treatment begins with motion in the head, neck, and trunk and should then branch into the extremities. This also supports the theory that stability must first be achieved proximally before <u>Fine motor</u> skills can be practiced distally.

• Early motor behavior is dominated by reflex activity. Mature motor behavior is supported or reinforced by postural reflexes (Voss, 1967). Reflexes that exist in the newborn and help a child develop eventually become integrated so that reflex behavior is not visible or evident. When voluntary movement is not possible, a person's nervous system can recall those reflexes to help achieve movement.

- Voluntary movement must involve the reversal of a particular action or movement (Voss, 1967). In order to have motor control both directions of movement must be practiced. For instance, a patient needs to be retrained on both how to dress and undress him or herself. Likewise, a patient who is practicing standing must also practice sitting.

- The growth of motor behavior has cyclic trends, as evidenced by shifts between flexor and extensor dominance (Voss, 1967). Balance must be achieved between antagonist muscle groups. For example, if a patient who has had a stroke demonstrates strong flexion, then extension should be emphasized during treatment.

- Developing motor behavior is expressed in an orderly sequence of total patterns of movement and posture. Treatment should incorporate a sequence of developmental positions (like that which infants go through during normal development: rolling, crawling, creeping, standing, and walking), which can facilitate movement. For instance, dressing can first be attempted while rolling, bridging, and going from supine to sit rather than beginning in a less stable sitting or standing position.

- Normal development does follow an orderly sequence; however, overlapping occurs (Voss, 1967). A child does not wait until he or she has mastered one activity before beginning another. Likewise during treatment, a patient does not wait to begin standing until he or she is able to sit perfectly.

- Movement depends on the balance and interaction

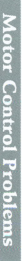

between antagonists (Voss, 1967). This is one of the main objectives of this approach and again reiterates the importance of strengthening the weaker motion of an extremity or the trunk. Voluntary movement will be difficult if one motion such as flexion dominates. If spasticity is demonstrated, then it will need to be inhibited prior to the facilitation of antagonist muscles.

- Improvement in motor ability depends on motor learning (Voss, 1967). The therapist should provide as many sensory inputs as possible such as verbal, tactile, and visual cues to help the patient relearn a task.
- Frequency of stimulation and repetitive activity are used to promote ad for retention of motor learning, and for the development of strength and endurance (Voss, 1967). The patient must practice for motor learning to occur, and for the action to become automatic.
- Goal-directed activities coupled with techniques of facilitation are used to hasten learning of total patterns of walking and <u>Self-care</u> activities (Voss, 1967). Facilitation should not occur independent of a purposeful task, but neither should a functional activity be practiced with any facilitation of normal movements or motions.

Treatment

- *Diagonal Patterns*: The use of diagonal patterns in treatment helps practice the movements used during functional activities. Each major body part performs two diagonal patterns, which include a flexion and extension component as well as a rotational component and abduction or adduction. To complete a diagonal pattern, add both components of each pattern together below; for example, the D_1 diagonal pattern happens when a patient uses both the flexion and extension components added together.

- Unilateral Patterns
  - *Upper Extremity D_1 Flexion (antagonist of D_1 extension)*: A pattern that includes scapula elevation, abduction, and rotation; shoulder flexion, adduction, and external rotation; elbow in flexion or extension; forearm supination; wrist flexion to the radial side; finger flexion and adduction; and thumb adduction. Functional examples include tennis forehand stroke or combing hair on the right side of the head with the left hand (or vice versa).
  - *Upper Extremity D_1 Extension (antagonist of D_1 flexion)*: A pattern that includes scapula depression, adduction, and rotation; shoulder extension, abduction, and internal rotation; elbow in flexion or extension; forearm pronation; wrist extension to the ulnar side; finger extension and abduction; and thumb in palmar abduction. Functional examples include tennis backhand stroke or pushing a car door open from the inside of the car.
  - *Upper Extremity D_2 Flexion (antagonist of D_2 extension)*: A pattern that includes scapula elevation, adduction, and rotation; shoulder flexion, abduction, and external rotation; elbow in flexion or extension; forearm supination; wrist extension to the radial side; finger extension and abduction; and thumb extension. Functional examples include the backstroke in swimming or combing hair on the right side of the head with the right hand.
  - *Upper Extremity D_2 Extension (antagonist of D_2 flexion)*: A pattern that includes scapula depression, abduction, and rotation; shoulder extension, adduction, and internal rotation; elbow in flexion or extension; forearm pronation; wrist flexion to the ulnar side; finger flexion and adduction; and thumb opposition. Functional examples include pitching a baseball or buttoning pants on the right side of the waist with the left hand.

- *Lower Extremity D_1 Flexion (antagonist of D_1 extension)*: A pattern that includes hip flexion, adduction, and external rotation; knee in flexion or extension; and ankle and foot dorsiflexion with inversion and toe extension. Functional examples include putting a shoe on with the leg crossed or kicking a ball.

- *Lower Extremity D_1 Extension (antagonist is D_1 flexion)*: A pattern that includes hip extension, abduction and internal rotation; knee in flexion or extension; and ankle and foot plantar flexion with eversion and toe flexion. Functional examples include placing the leg into pants or rolling from prone to supine.

- *Lower Extremity D_2 Flexion (antagonist of D_2 extension)*: A pattern that includes hip flexion, abduction, and internal rotation; knee in flexion or extension; and ankle and foot dorsiflexion with eversion and toe extension. Functional examples include a side karate kick or drawing the feet toward the bottom during the breaststroke in swimming.

- *Lower Extremity D_2 Extension (antagonist of D_2 flexion)*: A pattern that includes hip extension, adduction and external rotation; knee in flexion or extension; and ankle and foot plantar flexion with inversion and toe flexion. Functional examples include sitting on floor with legs extended and crossed, or the push-off in gait.

- Bilateral Patterns
  - *Symmetrical patterns*: These occur when both extremities move and complete the same patterns at the same time. These patterns are often the easiest to learn, and they also help facilitate or influence head, neck and trunk flexion/extension. Some examples would be D_1 extension while pushing off of a chair to stand up, D_2 extension while pulling a shirt off over the head, or D_2 flexion while lifting a large item off of a shelf overhead.

- *Asymmetrical patterns*. These occur when both extremities complete different patterns while moving toward the same side of the body. These help facilitate trunk rotation, and can occur in a chopping or lifting pattern when more rotation occurs. Some examples would be D_2 flexion to the left with the left arm and D_1 flexion to the left with the right arm while putting on a left earring, or D_2 extension to the left with the right arm and D_1 extension to the left with the left arm while zipping a side zipper on the left hip. A chopping pattern occurs with the arms in contact during the task. If chopping to the right, the right arm begins in D_1 flexion with the left hand gripping the wrist of the right arm. The right arm moves into D_1 extension with the left arm still grasping the right wrist and moving into D_2 extension. A lifting pattern also occurs with both arms in contact. If lifting to the left, the left arm begins in D_2 extension with the right hand gripping the wrist of the left arm. The left arm moves into D_2 flexion with the right arm still grasping the left wrist and moving into D_1 flexion.

- *Reciprocal patterns*: These occur when both extremities complete patterns in opposite directions at the same time. These help facilitate stabilization of the head, neck, and trunk, since they must remain in midline while each extremity moves outward. These can occur in any combination with the extremities moving in the same diagonal or different diagonals. Many functional activities occur in these patterns, such as donning a coat, walking, pitching a baseball, or swimming the sidestroke.

- *Total Patterns*: The use of total patterns helps facilitate diagonal patterns and also the interaction of the extremities with the trunk, neck, and head during movement. The therapist helps position the patient so that reflexes can help assist with the intended movement.

- *Prone-on-elbows*: The patient begins lying in prone with both lower extremities in symmetrical extension and the head at midline. The patient's arms are resting on the floor in D$_2$ flexion with the palmar surface of the hands on the floor slightly above the head. The therapist straddles the patient at the level of the patient's hips and applies Manual contacts to the patient's pectoral region with the therapist's fingers adducted and relaxed. After giving Verbal cues, the therapist leans back and gently pulls the patients shoulders posteriorly so that the patient's arms naturally pull medially until the patient is prone on elbows. The reflexes, which support this motion, include the optical and labyrinthine righting Reflexes and reactions.

- *Supine to side-lying*: The patient begins with the upper and lower extremities, which will be "up" after rolling onto his or her side, in D$_1$ flexion. The therapist sits on the side to which the patient is rolling toward and applies manual contacts to the patient's scapula and pelvis. With verbal cues, the patient log-rolls into side-lying with the therapist's assistance. The Reflex, which supports this motion, is the ATNR.

- *Side-lying to side-sitting*: The patient begins with both the upper and lower extremities in assymetrical flexion. The therapist sits behind the patient's hips and applies manual contacts to the patient's shoulder girdle, which is nearest, the floor. With verbal cues and assistance, the patient assumes a side-sitting position. The reflex, which supports this motion, is Body on body righting.

- *Supine to long sitting*: The patient begins with the lower extremities slightly abducted and symmetrically extended. The therapist straddles the patient at the level of the patient's knees and applies manual contacts to the dorsal surface of the patient's wrists. With verbal cues, the patient assumes a long sitting position. The reflexes, which support this motion, are optical and labyrinthine righting.

- *Prone to hands and knees*: The patient begins in prone with the hips flexed and the lower extremities slightly abducted. The therapist straddles the patient while placing the patient's hips between the therapist's knees. The therapist applies manual contacts to the patient's pectoral region while giving verbal cues for the patient to look up. The patient is then assisted into the hands and knees position. The <u>Reflex</u> that supports this motion is either the STNR (if patient's head is midline) or the ATNR (if patient's head is turned to one side).

- *Kneeling*: The patient begins either in hands and knees position or heel sitting. The therapist can either stand behind or in front of the patient depending on the patient's balance. The therapist applies manual contacts on the patient's pelvis and assists the patient into kneeling while giving verbal cues. The <u>Reflexes</u>, which support this motion, are optical and labyrinthine righting, and <u>Equilibrium reactions</u>.

- *Hands and knees to plantigrade*: The patient begins in the hands and knees position with the therapist applying manual contacts to the patient's pelvis. The therapist stands behind the patient. With verbal cues, the patient brings each foot forward into a flat position on the floor and stands, or the patient can simply straighten his or her knees. The reflexes, which support this motion, are optical and labyrinthine righting, and equilibrium reactions.

Techniques used during PNF. PNF superimposes these techniques on movement and posture (Voss, 1967; 1967; Voss, Iota, & Myers, 1985).

- Verbal cues can help reinforce movement.
- Visual cues help the patient identify the goal of the motion.
- Manual contacts refers to the therapist strategically placing his or her hands on the patient to provide pressure and sensory cues for facilitation. Contact should be given to reinforce the movement of the appropriate muscles completing the motion.
- Stretch is another facilitation method to help strengthen voluntary movement. Sherrington's principle (1961) states that a stretch to a muscle sends excitatory messages to the stretched muscle while sending inhibitory messages to the antagonistic muscle. During PNF treatment, the muscle to be facilitated should be stretched during a movement pattern when it is in its lengthened range of the pattern.
- Traction promotes movement by sending messages to the joint receptors while the joint surfaces are separated. Traction can specifically facilitate increase range of motion in painful joints.
- Approximation promotes stability by sending messages to the joint receptors while the joint surfaces are compressed. This technique can be applied during weight-bearing activities.
- Maximal resistance is the greatest amount of resistance, which can be given while a muscle contracts and/or completes its full range of motion without disrupting the movement or breaking an isometric contraction. The theory again is based on Sherrington's principle (1961) of irradiation, which states that stronger muscles can reinforce weaker ones. Resistance helps increase the patient's strength during the movement because the movement requires the patient's maximal effort.
- *Repeated contractions*, which are directed to the agonist, increase a patient's strength and endurance as well as provide the practice necessary for motor learning.

Motor Control Problems

- *Rhythmic initiation,* also directed to the agonist, provides sensory cues so that the patient feels a pattern before attempting to complete it. The therapist should first have the patient relax and passively complete the pattern. Then the patient should be asked to assist with the movement until he or she can actively complete it unassisted. Finally, the motion can be resisted to help strengthen the contraction.
- Reversal of antagonists may increase pain and spasticity, so these techniques may be contraindicated for some patients.
  - *Slow reversal* begins with an isotonic contraction of the antagonist against resistance followed by an isotonic contraction of the agonist against resistance. An isometric contraction at the end of the range following the above sequence is a technique called slow reversal-hold.
  - *Rhythmic stabilization* may be contraindicated for cardiac patients due to the tendency for the patient to hold his or her breath during this technique. Repeating isometric contractions increases stability. Resistance is placed against both agonist and antagonist muscles. The patient is asked to hold a contraction while resistance is given to the antagonist group. Then the patient is asked to continue holding while resistance is switched to the agonist muscle group. Switching from one group to another continues 3–4 repetitions without allowing the patient to rest.
- *Relaxation techniques* can help increase range of motion.
  - *Contact-relax* begins with an isotonic contraction against maximal resistance during the antagonistic pattern, allowing movement during only the rotational component of the pattern. Next, the patient relaxes while the therapist passively completes the agonistic part of the pattern. This is commonly used

184

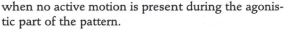

when no active motion is present during the agonistic part of the pattern.

- *Hold-relax* is similar to the above technique; however, an isometric contraction is completed during the antagonistic pattern, followed by relaxation and active movement during the agonistic pattern. This technique may be beneficial for a patient with RSD.

- *Slow-reversal-hold-relax* starts with an isotonic contraction. Next, the patient completes an isometric contraction, followed by relaxation of the antagonistic pattern. Finally, the patient actively moves through the agonistic pattern.

- *Rhythmic rotation* occurs while the therapist passively moves a part through a pattern. Whenever resistance or tone is felt against the movement, the part should be rotated slowly in one direction and then the other until relaxation occurs.

Neurodevelopmental Treatment, The Bobath Approach. This approach was specifically developed for patients with hemiplegia or Cerebral palsy, and the main goal is to train or retrain normal movement. In the case of the patient with hemiplegia, the patient's muscles are reeducated both as single units and as groups.

General Principles

- Movements that either increase abnormal muscle tone or facilitate abnormal movement patterns should be avoided.

- The goal is to produce normal movement or posture; however, treatment does not proceed in a developmental sequence. Rather, treatment should focus on movement that assists the patient with completing his or her functional activities.

- The patient's weak side should be included in all treatment so that functional use of the weak side becomes natural and also so that symmetry between the patient's extremities can be reestablished.

Motor Control Problems

- Treatment should demonstrate an improvement in the normal movement patterns and functional use of the patient's involved side.

Problem Areas in the Patient with Hemiplegia

- Normal movement patterns cannot be produced when abnormal tone exists. Normal <u>Muscle tone</u> exists when the muscle has enough strength to move a body part against gravity but does not change the speed of a normal movement or restrict the movement in any way. <u>Flaccidity</u> occurs when a patient has very low muscle tone and is not able to lift the body part against gravity. Low muscle tone usually occurs during the acute stage of the stroke and immediately following. As tone redevelops in the body part, <u>Spasticity</u> or very high tone may occur so that the patient cannot voluntarily move a body part against a very strong contraction in the <u>Antagonist</u> of the movement being attempted.

- A loss of postural control also inhibits normal movement. When completing activities, muscles automatically activate so that balance and equilibrium as well as stability at proximal joints occurs. The patient with hemiplegia can no longer rely on this automatic reaction of postural and stabilizing muscles, so he or she uses adaptive equipment such as a walker to compensate for this loss.

- Coordinated movements become difficult. When completing a motion, the patient's muscles may activate at the wrong time. Also, not all muscles required for a motion may have returned since the stroke; so only a few muscles may be trying to substitute and compensate in order to complete a task.

- All of the above deficits combine so that functional activities cannot be completed normally. The patient has difficulty coordinating the involved side with the noninvolved side while completing tasks.

Treatment Techniques

- *Weightbearing* on the affected extremity can have many positive effects. It can help normalize abnormal tone by either facilitating low tone or inhibiting high tone. It also provides the patient with sensory input and increases the patient's awareness of the affected extremity.

  - The patient can be positioned in bed so that he or she is lying on the affected side.

  - The patient should be encouraged to bear weight equally on both hips when sitting or feet when standing to complete activities.

  - The therapist can help position the affected upper extremity in a weightbearing position during reaching activities, which is especially helpful for those patients who demonstrate flexor synergy. Prior to weightbearing, the therapist should complete scapular mobilization to ensure that the scapula is gliding well. Also, the head of the humerus should be repositioned into the glenoid fossa if Subluxation has occurred.

    → The patient's affected hand should be placed on a chair or bench alongside the patient but far enough from the patient's hip so that the wrist is not hyperextended. The arm should be externally rotated (the hand is nearly perpendicular to the patient's trunk) and the elbow held in extension by the therapist. The elbow may be allowed to slightly flex; however the therapist should not allow the elbow to flex too much or the patient will not benefit from weightbearing through the shoulder. The patient should shift weight over the affected arm rather than "propping" him- or herself on the arm for extended periods of time, which could produce stress in the joints.

    → *Contraindications*: The patient should not complete

this activity if there is extreme pain or edema in the affected arm.

→ The patient can also complete weightbearing activities on the affected forearm which should be forward (0° of rotation) with the elbow flexed and the wrist in neutral.

- *Handling* occurs when the therapist directly facilitates or inhibits the patient's movements by placing his or her hands on the patient to provide normal alignment, complete normal movement patterns, or change abnormal tone. As the patient increases active movement, the therapist should lessen the amount of handling used.

  - Key points of control are the areas of the patient's body where the therapist can most effectively facilitate/inhibit movement, and they include the spine/rib cage, pelvis, shoulder, hand, and foot.

  - Hand placement depends on the type of movement completed as well as the amount of tone present. Firm pressure helps inhibit spasticity and abnormal patterns while light pressure facilitates active movement and steer the patient in the correct pattern of movement.

  - Inhibition techniques are used with patients who demonstrate spasticity or associated reactions. They include weight bearing, trunk rotation, and the lengthening of tight muscles (i.e., scapula mobilization, see below).

  - Facilitation techniques are used with patients who demonstrate either spasticity or flaccidity. They include the therapist guiding the patient through normal movement patterns, so that learning can occur and the patient can begin to actively assist with normal movement. If flaccidity is present, then Stimulation techniques, such as Tapping or Vibration, are used along with the facilitation techniques to help increase low tone.

- *Trunk rotation* can help the patient disassociate movements in the upper extremities from those in the lower extremities. Activities that strengthen the trunk muscles help the trunk to be a more stable foundation, and this allows the extremities to work without the patient needing to focus both on balance in the trunk as well as movement in the extremities. Trunk rotation also provides the patient with sensory input from and visual input toward the affected side.

- *Scapula mobilization* is the act of lengthening tight muscles around the scapula to prevent pain and maintain or increase upper extremity movement. This task is normally completed in supine, but it can be completed in side lying or sitting also. Mobilization begins with the patient's arm at his or her side. With the patient supine, the therapist sits on the patient's affected side. The therapist faces the patient and places his or her outermost hand on the patient's scapula and his or her innermost hand around the proximal part of the humerus. The lower part of the arm should be cradled into the therapist's elbow (the therapist must bend at the hips to achieve this position). While externally rotating the humerus to neutral, the therapist elevates/depresses and abducts/adducts the scapula. Once the scapula is gliding, the patient's shoulder can be flexed between 30° and 60° flexion and the same gliding motions completed. If the scapula again glides well and the patient does not have pain, the shoulder can be flexed greater (up to 90°) and the same motions completed. Once the scapula has demonstrated these motions, passive range of motion of the shoulder can be completed. *Precaution*: Care should be taken that the humerus is externally rotated to neutral during shoulder flexion and abduction above 60° so that the head of the humerus can clear the acromion process. Otherwise, the patient may complain of pain from the impingement of the supraspinatus tendon, or full motion will not be achieved.

- *Scapular protraction* is the first step in disassociating the components of the flexor synergy. The therapist should place one hand on the medial border of the scapula while gently holding the patient's arm in the other hand. The arm and scapula should gently be guided forward and held in a protracted position for a few seconds. The arm should then be allowed to slide back into retraction, but the therapist should never assist the arm back into retraction.

- *Place and hold* activities allow the therapist to gradually withdraw assistance from movement. The patient is guided through movement by the therapist and then asked to hold a particular position (such as 90° flexion or slight abduction). At first, the therapist is not able to withdraw all assistance; instead the assistance is decreased from maximal to moderate assistance. The therapist then assists the arm to its original position. As active movement increases, the goal is for the patient to place and hold the arm in the expected position without assistance.

- *Reducing a Subluxation* must be completed prior to passive range of motion of the affected arm. The therapist first upwardly rotates the affected scapula. Then the therapist firmly grasps the proximal humerus while pushing it upward into the glenoid fossa and externally rotating it to neutral. After repositioning the humerus, the therapist can complete passive movements of the patient's arm with one hand while maintaining the head of the humerus in the fossa with the other hand.

- *Position pelvis forward* means to assist the patient so that he she is sitting with the pelvis in a neutral position rather than in posterior pelvic tilt, which often occurs after a stroke. A posterior pelvic tilt can help

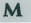

facilitate flexor synergy as well as cause swallowing and safety problems, since the patient appears he or she is going to slide out of a chair when sitting. The therapist can have the patient practice bending forward toward his or her shoes so that the inhibition of the extensor synergy occurs at the hip, as well as the promotion of symmetrical weightbearing through both feet and scapular protraction.

- *Slow, controlled movements* prevent high tone. Quick movements facilitate tone and flexor synergy; therefore, they should be avoided.
- The therapist should give feedback, so that the patient can learn which movements are normal and which are compensatory or substitutions.
- *Proper Positioning* helps prevent synergies and compensatory movements also.
  - Bed Positioning
    - → Lying on the affected side helps provide input through weightbearing. The patient should be positioned with the head symmetrical; a pillow may be used if the head is not flexed too much. Next, the affected arm should be fully protracted and flexed at the shoulder to at least 90° with the elbow flexed and the forearm supinated so that the affected hand is under the pillow. The elbow may also be extended with the wrist slightly off the bed to help encourage wrist extension. The affected leg should be extended at the hip and slightly flexed at the knee, while the unaffected leg is supporting on a pillow in hip and knee flexion for comfort. This position is preferred for patients with Hemiplegia.
    - → Lying on the nonaffected side begins with the head positioned symmetrically on a pillow. Again, the affected shoulder is fully protracted and flexed to 90°. The affected arm should be

supported on a pillow so that the wrist is placed in neutral and not allowed to flex. A pillow should also support the affected leg so that the hip and knee are flexed, and the foot and ankle are supported so that the foot does not invert.

→ Lying supine begins with the head symmetrical. A pillow should be placed under the affected shoulder so that it is symmetrical with the non-affected shoulder; however, care should be taken so that it is not overly raised since this could result in anterior subluxation. The affected arm should be extended and supinated with a pillow supporting the entire arm.

• When sitting, the patient should have the hips at 90° flexion, the knees and ankles less than but near 90° flexion, the trunk upright, the head at midline, and the affected arm supported.

• Whenever possible, therapy should occur while the patient is either sitting in a straight-backed chair or standing rather than sitting in a wheelchair.

• *Bilateral clasped activities* allow the nonaffected arm to help retrain normal movement patterns in the affected arm. Again, the nonaffected arm provides sensory input and increases the patient's awareness of the affected arm.

• *Guiding* occurs when the therapist places his or her hand on the patient's arm and helps move it through normal movement patterns.

• *Room arrangement* also helps encourage the patient to look toward the affected side rather than allowing the patient to neglect that side. The bed should be turned so that the patient must look toward the affected side to see persons entering the room. Chairs for visitors should be placed on the patient's affected side. The telephone or television should also be positioned on the patient's affected side to encourage awareness of the affected side. The patient's call light should *not* be placed on the affected side, since a patient with profound neglect may never find the call light on the affected side.

- *Dressing technique* should be completed in a straight-back chair if possible rather than on the edge of the bed. The patient should attempt to involve both the affected and the nonaffected extremities in the activity, and the therapist should always sit on the patient's affected side. The patient dons a shirt by placing it with the armhole and sleeve for the affected arm between his or her knees. The patient then bends forward to place the arm into the sleeve; this helps disrupt the extension synergy of the lower extremity and the flexion synergy of the upper extremity. The patient completes the activity by dressing the nonaffected side. When completing lower extremity dressing, the patient should use bilateral clasped hands to help the affected leg cross over the nonaffected leg (the therapist can assist as needed). The patient then uses the nonaffected arm to put the pants or sock/shoe on the affected leg first, and completes the activity by dressing the nonaffected side.

Movement Therapy of Brunnstrom. (Brunnstrom, 1970, 1996). A traditional approach to the treatment of persons with motor control problems, specifically patients who have had a stroke/CVA. This type of treatment is based on the theory that redevelopment of motor control should proceed along the same line that normal motor development proceeds. from reflexive behavior to voluntary movement. Other important principles include the following: treatment should focus on the quality of the movement itself, and motor control redevelops in a proximal to distal sequence. See <u>Motor control problems</u> and <u>Movement therapy of Brunnstrom</u> for a more complete discussion of the theories and techniques of this treatment.

Multidisciplinary Team. Professionals from various disciplines who assess and treat clients autonomously and meet regularly to coordinate treatment.

Multi-infarct Dementia. A condition that results in impaired cognition from multiple sites of damage due to vascular disease. This form of organic brain disease can cause a rapid decline in mental ability.

Multiple Personality Disorder. The presence of two or more personalities that are distinct and can alternate in certain situations. Each personality is usually not aware of the other personalities. Treatment goal is to help the individual gain insight into the origins, needs, and problems that are produced by these multiple personalities. Creative arts and insight therapy are effective.

Multiple Sclerosis. A disease of the nervous system that results in demyelination of nerve fibers in the white matter of the spinal cord and brain. After demyelination occurs, sclerotic patches form to create lesions. This disorder occurs in exacerbations and remissions, which cause a fluctuation in a patient's function. The cause is unknown; however, some possible causes include decreased blood flow, vitamin deficiency, autoimmune reaction, a slow-acting virus, allergies, and trauma. Onset occurs in persons between the ages of 20–40 years of age, and women are 50% more likely to incur this disease.

Specific Treatments
- Complete resistive strengthening activities, but do not cause fatigue
- Maintain coordination and reduce tremors by using weighted objects for activities or placing light weights on the wrists
- Improve the patient's endurance through exercise and rest, which are alternated to prevent fatigue
- Fabricate splints or provide stretch to tight muscles to prevent deformity

(sidebar) Multiple Sclerosis

- Instruct the patient on the importance of skin inspection to prevent pressure sores if the patient demonstrates <u>Sensory deficits</u>
- Increase the patient's ability to use tactile or other sensory cues if vision is failing
- Educate the patient on energy conservation and work simplification techniques
- Address safety and memory concerns by establishing reminders such as routines or tools like notebooks, signs, etc.
- Teach the patient <u>Stress management</u> and <u>Relaxation techniques</u>
- Encourage the patient to join a support group for socialization
- Assist the patient with adjustment to the disease by setting realistic goals
- Recommend assistive devices to increase independence with Self-care activities and equipment to increase safety and mobility in home
- Explore leisure and job interests as needed or help retrain skills to allow return to previous leisure and work activities

Contraindications/Precautions

- Expect some loss of function following an exacerbation. a remission does not mean that all function will return exactly like it was prior to the exacerbation

Muscle Strength. Neuromusculoskeletal ability that indicates the degree of muscle power when lifting objects, resisting force, or maintaining posture. Muscle weakness can occur in <u>Multiple sclerosis</u>, <u>Parkinson's disease</u>, <u>Muscular dystrophy</u>, <u>Stroke</u>, and other neuromuscular diseases. Treatment to increase muscle strength include <u>Graded activities</u> and <u>Isometric exercises</u> such as weight lifting (Kendall, McCreary, & Provance, 1993). See <u>Appendix D</u>.

Muscle Tone. Neuromusculoskeletal component that indicates a muscle's degree of tension at rest or resistance in

Muscle Tone. *(continued)*

response to stretch. Hypertonicity or spasticity indicates high abnormal tone while hypotonicity or flaccidity indicates low muscular tone or tension. Abnormal muscle tone is one of the symptoms in children with <u>Cerebral palsy</u>; <u>Neurodevelopmental treatment</u> is applied to reduce spasticity. It is assessed by measuring the amount of tension in the fibers of a muscle, or the amount of resistance in the muscle when it is stretched. Slight resistance can be felt in a muscle with normal tone when it is stretched. <u>Facilitation</u> and <u>Inhibition techniques</u> can be used to help increase or decrease muscle tone (Nichols, 1996).

Music Therapy.   Use of music for relaxation by creating an emotional climate, increasing movements in the client or the instruction on how to play a musical instrument. Psychological goals, for example, can be used to increase self-esteem or decrease depressive thoughts. Music therapy sessions include singing, rhythmic movement where the client moves to the music, listening to music that can be relaxing or stimulating to the client, or playing a musical instrument. The goals for music therapy are individualized. Although music therapy is an established profession, many occupational therapists incorporate a music program in treatment.

Myofacial Release.   A method for treating myofacial pain that considers both the origin of the pain and the resulting dysfunction. The three aspects of this approach include manual therapy, movement and exercise, and patient education. A whole body "hands-on" approach is used to release soft tissue (muscle) from abnormal grip of tight fascial (connective tissue).

Myasthenia Gravis.   A chronic and progressive disorder that results in weakness of the voluntary muscles. Weakness is characterized by exacerbations and remissions. This disorder most likely occurs from an autoimmune cause, and onset is more prevalent in women if the person is between 20–30 years of age. When comparing the incidence after age 40, this disorder occurs equally in men and women.

Specific Treatments

- Complete nonresistive activities to maintain ROM, strength, and endurance
- Apply equipment such as suspension slings or mobile arm supports to assist with weak voluntary movement
- Assist the patient in establishing a time management program so that activity is spread throughout the day and completed when the patient has the most energy
- Instruct the patient on energy conservation and work simplification principles
- Teach safe transfer methods using equipment as needed
- Educate the patient on Stress management and Relaxation techniques
- Encourage socialization, but remind the patient of the importance of frequent rest breaks to avoid fatigue
- Demonstrate assistive devices that can increase the patient's independence with Self-care activities
- Recommend techniques and diet consistency to increase the patient's ability to chew and swallow
- Provide recommendations concerning the modification of home or the work site to increase the patient's productivity and safety
- Explore new leisure interests as needed

Contraindications/Precautions

- Avoid overexertion and fatigue
- Monitor respiration
- Do not complete resistive activities
- Avoid the use of materials or activities that can exacerbate difficulty with breathing; for example, certain cleaning chemicals or sawdust from sanding wood should be avoided.

Narcissistic Personality Disorder.   An individual who
shows signs of grandiosity toward self, fantasies of power
over others, omniscience, self-importance, vanity, and a
strong need for admiration by others and opportunities for
exhibiting self. Sometimes the individual shows a lack of
empathy and understanding toward others. Group therapy
is effective to help the individual gain consensual validation
of behavior and to develop compassion for others. Reality
therapy has also been successful.

Naturopathy.   Based on a therapeutic system that does not
advocate the use of drugs. The naturopath employs natural
forces such as light, heat, air, water, massage, herbs, healthy
food, and vitamins in treating individuals with a dysfunction.

Neck Righting.   See Reflexes and reactions.

Negative Symptoms.   Losses or lessening of human functions such as the loss of motivation, withdrawal from social
interactions, apathy, flattening of affect, loss of words to
say, and loss of critical thinking or problem solving ability
such as in making decisions. Negative symptoms are associated with Schizophrenia.

Neurodevelopmental Treatment (Bobath).   A traditional approach to the treatment of persons with motor
control problems, specifically patients with hemiplegia or
Cerebral palsy. This approach states that treatment should
focus on the goal of movement and increasing the patient's
ability to complete his or her functional activities. Other
basic principles include the following: motor control redevelops in a proximal to distal sequence, and reflexes should
not be used to assist the patient with active movement. See
Motor control problems, Neurodevelopmental treatment
for further discussion of treatment.

Neuroma.   A mass of nerve fibers that forms alongside a
nerve, often near a laceration site.

Neuromuscular Electrical Stimulation (NMES).   A physical agent modality that uses electrical current to help reeducate and/or strengthen muscles, gain ROM, and reduce spasticity through the stimulation of antagonist muscles (DeVahl, 1992). See Physical agent modalities for further discussion and treatment.

Neurosis.   A term that was first defined in the DSM-I (American Psychiatric Association, 1952) as psychoneurotic and referred to behaviors in individuals marked by anxiety, avoidance, feelings of inadequacy, phobias, unhappiness, excessive guilt, and obsessive behavior. Currently in the DSM-IV (American Psychiatric Association, 1994) these behaviors are indicative of personality disorders.

Neutral Warmth.   A technique used to inhibit high Muscle tone. The patient is wrapped in a blanket for 5 to 10 minutes until the heat reaches the temperature center of the hypothalamus, which helps the patient relax. See Motor control problems, Rood approach for further discussion of inhibition techniques.

Nystagmus.   Involuntary eye movement, which can occur in a horizontal or vertical direction, that can cause balance problems and difficulty with postural alignment. Lesions of the vestibular system, brainstem, or cerebellum may result in involuntary nystagmus.

Object Permanence. A cognitive process in which infants (approximately 9 months) develop the concept that objects exist even if they are not in the child's line of vision.

Objective Psychological Test. A standardized test that contains comparative norms for interpreting individual raw scores.

Obsessive-Compulsive Personality Disorder. An individual who has a morbid concern with neatness, orderliness, perfection, and ritualistic or repetitive behavior. Symptoms include extreme preoccupation with details that interferes with task completion, excessive time at work at the expense of leisure, overconscientiousness regarding ethical or legal standards, lack of flexibility in decision making, a miserly spending attitude, and the hoarding of objects. Treatment includes Relaxation therapies, Stress management, and Paradoxical intention where the client learns how to control the behavior through self-regulation. Reduction of the general anxiety accompanying the behavior will usually reduce the obsession or compulsiveness. Bringing humor into a client's life is also important to some clients who categorize their behavior or thoughts as catastrophic.

Occupational Stress. The sum of the factors in the work environment that negatively affect the individual's psychophysiological adjustment or Homeostasis.

Occupational Therapy. The application of purposeful activities to prevent disability and injury in individuals who are at risk and to develop independence and restore functions in individuals who are disabled. Functional activities include the ability to Work, to be independent in Self-care, to engage in Leisure activities and to be effective in social interactions. The effectiveness of occupational therapy will depend on the therapist's ability to establish a therapeutic relationship and to select a purposeful activity that is meaningful to the client in producing a desired outcome.

Occupations.   The culturally and personally meaningful and purposeful activities that humans engage in during their everyday lives. These occupations include the major functions of life such as <u>Work</u>, <u>Leisure</u>, play, <u>Self-care</u>, rest, sleep, and social interactions.

Oculomotor Function.   Movement of the eye ball which is caused by the muscles attached to the eye. See <u>Appendix D</u> for specific muscles. The four parts of oculomotor function include range of motion, pursuits, convergence, and alignment.

- *Range of motion.* A test should be completed to check that all six extraocular muscles of the eye are able to contract and move the eye through its full available range. This is tested by holding a pencil in front of the patient and moving the pencil in a large H-pattern. The patient should follow the pencil with eye movements without moving his or her head.
- *Pursuits*. The ability to track objects, or scan, is another component of oculomotor function which is tested. The therapist should move a pencil while asking the patient to follow the movement with his or her eyes.
- *Convergence*. A test should also be completed to check the ability of the eyes to focus on an object in close proximity. Measurement should be taken at the closest point of vision with *both* eyes. The therapist should slowly move a pencil toward the patient's nose and take note of the point of convergence, which is normally 6 to 8 inches from the person's nose. The eyes will track the pencil together to the closest point of focus, but then one eye will drift while the other eye continues to track the object.
- *Alignment*. The final test of oculomotor function checks that both eyes are being used when viewing an object. The therapist should use the corneal light reflex by asking the patient to look at a penlight held 12 inches in front of the patient's eyes. The therapist should observe a reflection in the same location on the cornea of both eyes.

- Oculomotor function, <u>Visual acuity</u>, and <u>Visual fields</u> comprise the visual foundation skills which may decrease perception or negatively affect a test of perception. See <u>Cognitive-perceptual deficits</u> for further discussion and treatment of perceptual problems.

Olfactory Sensation. Receiving, distinguishing, localizing, and interpreting odors and smells through the nose. Damage to the olfactory mechanism will affect taste.

On-the-Job Evaluations. Situations in which the client is evaluated while employed.

Open Reduction. The act of correcting a fracture through surgical intervention. During surgery, hardware, such as rods and screws, are attached to the bone to help maintain alignment while the bone heals. The hardware is internal, which is referred to as an internal fixator. A patient who has undergone this procedure has a diagnosis of ORIF, or open reduction internal fixator.

Operant Conditioning. Behavior therapy in which an individual's positive behavior is reinforced and negative behavior is not reinforced. Behavior is shaped by reinforcing sequential steps in a hierarchical manner.

Opposition. A motion that combines thumb flexion and abduction with medial rotation of the CMC joints and flexion of the MCP joint in order to bring the <u>Palmar surfaces</u> of the distal phalanxes of the thumb and each finger into contact. It should be noted that the *tip* of the thumb and each finger can achieve contact without having to perform opposition.

Optical Righting. See <u>Reflexes and reactions</u>.

Oral-Motor Control. The ability to coordinate the musculature around the mouth, tongue, lips, and palate in performing activities such as eating, speaking, singing, sucking through a straw, or playing a musical instrument such as the oboe.

Orientation. A cognitive component indicating an individual's awareness and understanding of person, place, time, and situation. An item in an orientation test will ask the client to state who he or she is, where one is, the year it is, and why the individual is in a hospital or care center. See Cognitive-perceptual deficits for further discussion and treatment.

Orthomolecular Medicine. The study of the relationship between vitamins in the body and the onset of diseases such as the relationship between B-complex vitamins and psychiatric disorders. Orthomolecular practitioners recommend megadoses of vitamins in treating specific psychiatric disorders.

Orthosis. An external device which is attached to a patient's body or used by the patient to help restore function (Tan, 1998). Orthoses may be used to (a) decrease the effect of abnormal muscle tone, (b) support a weak extremity, (c) immobilize an extremity following surgery or trauma, or (d) correct deformity. Orthoses that are applied to hands are often referred to as Splints. The category of splints may be further subdivided into static and dynamic splints. *Static splints* have no moving parts, so they are used for support and stability. The therapist fabricates a static splint to immobilize a joint or prevent contractures and/or deformity. *Dynamic splints* have moving parts, which are used to assist in the proper alignment of fractures, substitute for muscles that have undergone surgical repair, increase ROM and decrease contractures, or control movement. The therapist fabricates a dynamic splint to increase mobility at a joint. Other types of orthoses include *cervical collars* to prevent neck flexion; *back braces* to prevent curvature of the spine or to support weak musculature; *arm slings* to support the shoulder joint; *braces* to support the foot, which are often referred to as ankle-foot orthoses; *hinge splints* which are artificially powered to provide movement;

Orthosis. *(continued)*
and suspension slings or mobile arm supports to assist if
muscle contraction is weak and movement is difficult. See
Appendix C.

Orthostatic Hypotension. A condition of dizziness, nausea, or loss of consciousness from rapidly changing positions.
This most often occurs when a person has been lying down or
sitting for an extended period of time, which can allow blood
to pool in the lower extremities or abdomen. When the
patient then stands, blood pressure decreases rapidly and
causes the above symptoms. A patient may be placed in a
reclined position until the symptoms diminish. Some medications place a patient at higher risk for hypotension.

Osteoarthritis. A disorder characterized by a loss of hya-
line cartilage or changes in subchondral bone, which can
affect one or many joints. This disorder is also referred to as
degenerative joint disease. Osteoarthritis may be classified
as primary or secondary. *Primary osteoarthritis* usually occurs
due to genetic factors; whereas *secondary osteoarthritis* may
occur from trauma, inflammation, endocrine and metabolic
diseases, congenital or developmental defects, or prolonged
occupational stress. Onset can begin as early as 20–30 years
of age; however, most people suffer from this disorder by
70 years of age.
Specific treatments
- Apply paraffin or other thermal modalities prior to ROM
  activities to help increase range
- Fabricate Splints to prevent deformity and increase functional use of the hands. Splints that may be useful include
  the wrist cock-up splint, resting hand splint, thumb spica
  splint, or finger gutter splints
- Complete activities to increase strength of muscles surrounding the affected joints
- Teach joint protection principles and remind the patient
  to use these techniques during activities

- Instruct the patient on pain management techniques
- Educate the patient on energy conservation and work simplification techniques
- Help the patient organize the home to make items more accessible and reduce barriers to mobility and function
- Encourage the patient to join a support group for socialization
- Retrain Self-care activities by using techniques and devices that can reduce the stress on joints
- Complete a home evaluation and modify equipment to make tasks simpler, for example, elevate a chair or the bed for easier transfers
- Suggest that the patient purchase and wear clothing that is easy to don and doff, for example, a female patient can purchase a more elastic sports bra and don it overhead if she is unable to hook a brassiere
- Encourage the continuation of job and leisure activities, but with utilization of new methods to decrease stress on joints

Contraindications/Precautions

- Avoid overexertion
- Monitor skin for redness if splints are being used
- Ask the patient to avoid positions in bed that can lead to deformity such as a prone position or the use of many pillows

Outcome. The result of a treatment intervention. Outcomes research is the investigation of treatment methods in producing desired outcomes such as the decrease of negative symptoms in individuals with Schizophrenia.

Outcome Measure. A specific test, procedure, or tool that is used to measure the results of a treatment intervention. For example, an outcome measure for pain is the *McGill-Melzack Pain Inventory*.

Osteoarthritis

Paget's Disease. A condition that results in increased reabsorption and formation of bone, which causes softening and thickening of bones.

Pain Management. A holistic approach to treating chronic pain that takes into account the physiological, psychological, and cultural and spiritual aspects of the patient. Physical agent modalities, Stress management, Counseling and Psychotherapy, Support groups, and Biofeedback are used.

Pain Response. A perceptual process that enables an individual to identify and localize tissue damage, physiological changes such as extreme temperature, and psychological or emotional stress. Acute pain is usually a warning sign of sudden change such as a torn ligament or headache from emotional stress. Chronic pain that is continuous may have systemic symptoms affecting sleep, movement, gastrointestinal tract, and personality. Occupational therapists can treat pain through Stress management, Biofeedback, Splinting, Physical agent modalities, Arts and crafts, Relaxation training, and Support groups.

Palmar Prehension. Also referred to as the three-jaw chuck pinch, this pattern combines opposition and rotation of the thumb with flexion of the index and long fingers for pad-to-pad contact of the fingers and thumb. This pattern is used when tying shoelaces or picking small objects up off of a flat surface.

Palpation. The therapist uses the pads of his or her fingers (usually the index and long fingers) to feel bony landmarks, muscle contractions, or tone. This technique is important when finding landmarks for goniometer placement during measurement of ROM and is essential in detecting a muscle contraction when the muscle is not strong enough to produce movement. Also, it is important to palpate a muscle while it contracts to ensure there is no substitution being made to complete a motion. See <u>Appendix G</u> for common substitutions for motions.

Palmar Grasp Reflex.   See <u>Reflexes and reactions</u>.

Panic Disorder.   An anxiety disorder characterized by panic attacks and accompanied by acute anxiety, terror or fright, hyperventilation, sweating, chest pain, dizziness, and a feeling of losing control of self. Panic attacks can occur suddenly and last for minutes with a sense of imminent danger or impending disaster. A panic disorder can lead to agoraphobia (fear of being in public and being alone). Treatment of this disorder includes <u>Cognitive-behavioral techniques</u> in which the individual learns how to self-regulate symptoms. Specific techniques include <u>Paradoxical intention</u>, <u>Desensitization</u>, and <u>Relaxation therapies</u>.

Paradigm.   A conceptual model that becomes universally accepted. For example, during the age of institutionalization (1920–1950) in the United States, the paradigm for treating mental illness was through hospitalization. In the 1960s, a shift in the paradigm occurred by the community mental health movement.

Paradoxical Intention (Frankl, 1967).   A behavior therapy technique based on the theory that individuals develop fears and tensions because of anticipatory <u>Anxiety</u>. In using this technique, the individual is told to think of something he fears most or to create a negative emotion such as anxiety. By creating a negative feeling, the individual begins to cognitively control the symptom. It has been used as a successful technique with those who stutter who consciously produce stuttering and by doing so to control the speech.

Paraffin.   A physical agent modality that uses conduction to transfer heat to superficial physiological tissue. See <u>Physical agent modalities</u> for further discussion and treatment.

Paraffin Therapy   is the application of hot wax, usually to the hand and fingers, to relieve pain such as in <u>Rheumatoid</u>

Paraffin Therapy. *(continued)*
or Osteoarthritis. Precautions should be noted when there are any skin infections.

Paranoid Personality Disorder. Marked by extreme suspiciousness and distrust of others. An individual with this disorder attributes hidden motives and agendas of hostility directed by others toward self. The individual is easily offended, tends to misread and distort verbal and nonverbal communications, and is hypervigilant. Treatment is based on the assumption that the client is harboring much anger that needs to be channeled into socially acceptable behaviors. Anger management, expressive arts, Stress management and Relaxation therapy has been shown to be effective

Paranoid Schizophrenia. A subcategory of Schizophrenia characterized by delusions, irrational beliefs, excessive suspicion, and feeling of persecutions by others.

Paraplegia. Paralysis of both lower extremities, usually due to a spinal injury.

Parataxic Distortion. The "uncommunicative, unintelligible, and misleading statements in allegedly communicative interpersonal contexts" (Sullivan, 1963, p. 23).

Paresthesia. The condition of feeling a "burning" or "pins and needles" sensation.

Parkinson's Disease. A degenerative disorder of the central nervous system, specifically the basal ganglia. Symptoms include Cogwheel rigidity, Bradykinesia, Akinesia, and impaired posture. Onset most commonly occurs after 40 years of age, and the cause is unknown.
Specific Treatments
- Complete activities to maintain ROM, especially extension
- Provide stretch to tight muscles to prevent contractures
- Use repetitive tasks to improve dexterity and coordination

- Remind the patient to continue reciprocal arm movements, moderate-sized steps, and initiation of ambulation
- Use music, singing, and dancing to assist with initiation of movement
- Treat motor planning and movement, especially trunk rotation, through the application of PNF patterns
- Cue the patient to check balance and posture and use self-correcting techniques when possible
- Complete a home evaluation and remove barriers to mobility
- Provide beat or rhythm through the use of a metronome or music while teaching balance and posture skills
- Instruct the patient on energy conservation and work simplification techniques
- Educate the patient on the disease process and expectations for therapy
- Teach the patient to use inhibition techniques to help normalize increased muscle tone
- Train the patient to use relaxation techniques as a means for also decreasing high tone
- Encourage the patient and family to join a support group
- Ask the patient to verbalize often during treatment to help maintain volume of the voice
- Teach the patient compensatory techniques to help maintain independence with Self-care activities if the patient demonstrates tremors. positioning the arms close to the body may help with stability during feeding, or stabilizing the arms on a table surface or the lap can help control tremors
- Explore job and leisure interests as needed

Contraindications/Precautions
- Stand near the patient when the patient is standing or walking, as there is an increased risk for loss of balance which can result in falls
- Observe the patient for symptoms that may result as side effects from medication

Parkinson's Disease

Parkinson's Disease

- Monitor the patient for signs of Depression

Partial Hospitalization. Includes day, evening, night and weekend day treatment programs for individuals who need a supportive environment during a period of crisis but are able to avoid hospitalization and to stay in the community.

Passive-Aggressive Personality Disorder. Characterized by stubbornness, procrastination, indecisiveness, envy, and resistance to requests and demands from others. An individual with this disorder tends not to be overtly hostile, but through indecision and defiance, creates negative confrontations with others. A psychodynamic approach using expressive and creative media is effective in helping the client resolve feelings.

Passive Range of Motion (PROM). The amount of movement at a joint when the joint is moved through its range by an outside force, rather than by the muscles that act on that joint. The abbreviation commonly used is PROM. A therapist often passively moves body parts through range to help prevent stiffness and contractures when the muscles are too weak. If only one extremity demonstrates limited ROM, then the therapist should compare to the unaffected extremity to determine the amount of impairment. If this is not possible, the therapist should refer to a table of average ranges, which can be found in Appendix E. For *contraindications/precautions* to ROM/measurement and specifics on measurement, see Range of motion.

Pelvic Tilt. A term used to refer to the position of the pelvis and its relationship to the spine. A patient's pelvis can demonstrate a posterior or anterior pelvic tilt. A patient who demonstrates *posterior pelvic tilt* appears to sit on the lower part of the sacrum, which makes the person look like he or she may slide out of the chair. The pelvis is tipped backward with the anterior superior iliac spines and the posterior superior iliac spines tilted more posteriorly than normal. Flexion of the spine results to help the patient keep the head upright, which may result in a concave curvature of the spine know as Kyphosis. A patient who demonstrates *anterior pelvic tilt* has the pelvis tipped forward with the anterior superior iliac spines down and the posterior superior iliac spines tilted more anteriorly than normal. Hyperextension of the spine allows the patient to remain upright, but this may result in a convex curvature of the spine known as Lordosis.

Perception.   The ability to gather sensory information and apply it within a meaningful framework of knowledge to help assign meaning to the sensory input. For example, a patient with intact spatial relations is able to feel his or her body position but then applies that to his or her existing knowledge of directions such as over, under, above, and so on to determine body position. See Cognitive-perceptual deficits for further discussion and treatment.

Perceptual Deficits.   See Cognitive-perceptual deficits for discussion and treatment.

Performance Areas of the Uniform Terminology. The occupations of daily life and include Activities of daily living, Work and productivity, and Play or Leisure.

Performance Components of the Uniform Terminology.   The fundamental human abilities that underlie the Performance areas. These include Sensorimotor, Cognitive integration, Psychosocial skills, and Psychological components.

Performance Contexts.   The temporal and environmental factors that influence an individual's abilities such as age, Developmental stages of life, severity of disabilities, physical environment, social network, and cultural aspects.

Performance Test.   A measure of an individual's skill or capacity such as grip strength, Range of motion, manual dexterity, or driving skills.

Peripheral.   See <u>Anatomical position</u>.

Peripheral Nerve Injuries.   Different nerve injuries result in different deformities. An ulnar nerve injury or palsy may cause the patient to have a <u>Claw hand</u>. A radial nerve injury or palsy can result in wrist drop.

Treatment

- Depending on which branches are injured, either or both sensory and motor reeducation may be necessary to the affected area.

- Sensory reeducation should be started as soon as possible. The patient can rub various textures over the affected area, or immerse the affected part into containers of different textured materials. For a more complete description of this treatment technique, see <u>Sensory deficits</u>, <u>Treatment</u>.

- The affected part may need to be immobilized for 3–5 weeks to allow some healing of the nerve, depending on the severity of the injury. Motor reeducation may begin following immobilization in the form of gentle active and passive range of motion to decrease stiffness.

- A <u>Splint</u> may be necessary to help oppose the agonist muscles since nerve damage can result in paralysis of antagonist muscles. For example, a patient with a radial nerve injury could get a contracture in wrist flexion since the wrist extension muscles are not able to oppose the strong wrist flexors.

- <u>Neuromuscular electrical stimulation</u> is used in some cases to assist the patient with the paralyzed or weak motion and to help prevent atrophy of muscles.

Personality Disorders.   Comprise a number of disorders including antisocial, histrionic, paranoid, passive-aggressive, obsessive-compulsive, schizoid, narcissistic, borderline, and avoidant types. The disorder usually begins during childhood or adolescence and continues into adulthood. Many times the disorder leads to self-defeating behaviors that interfere with the individual's ability to adapt to changes in the environment and to meet societal expectations.

Personality. The complex of characteristics, behavioral traits, and attitudes that distinguish an individual from others.

Pet Therapy. The therapeutic use of pets, to create an animal-human bond, which may improve a patient's physical and emotional health.

Phenomenological. The subjective experiences and feelings of an individual. Depressed feelings and delusions in an individual with mental illness can be considered phenomenological symptoms.

Phobia. An abnormal fear or irrational dread of a specific object (e.g., spiders), activity, (e.g., flying), or situation (e.g., being in an open plain).

Phonophoresis. The application of ultrasound in conveying medication into a tissue such as in Pain management. See Physical agent modalities for further discussion and treatment.

Physical Agent Modalities (PAMs). Therapeutic agents that use physical energy to promote physiological change in body tissue for the purpose of enhancing the treatment of occupation (Cameron, 1999). In using PAMS the therapist applies electrical stimulation, Massage, sound frequencies, hot or cold temperatures, vibration and joint manipulation to the patient. Examples are TENS (Gersh, 1992), Paraffin therapy, Hydrotherapy, Phonophoresis, Cryotherapy, Cranio-sacral therapy, and Ultrasound. Therapists using PAMs should have specialized training and/or certification in the use of the modality and the applications may be limited based on state laws and practice acts. AOTA recommends that an occupational therapist may use PAMS prior to or during treatment, providing that the main focus

Physical Agent Modalities (PAMs)

Physical Agent Modalities (PAMs). *(continued)*
of treatment is functional activities. The therapist must also
demonstrate knowledge of the theory, purpose, and techni-
cal skills required by the modality being used. PAMS are
also classified into two major categories: thermal modalities
and electrical modalities.

Thermal Modalities (Michlovitz, 1990a).

Heat. Heat is used to help decrease stiffness and pain,
increase soft tissue movement and range of motion,
relieve spasms, and assist with the reabsorption of
chronic edema. Collagen fibers will resist the temporary effects of stretch; however, heat can assist with
permanent relaxation of collagen fibers if applied
prior to prolonged stretch (such as splinting). Tissue
may be raised to a temperature of 105°–113° F. in
order to receive the optimal effects from heat; however heat above that may result in tissue damage.
Heat can be transferred through conduction, convection, or conversion.

Cold. Cold is used to help decrease pain and muscle
spasm; reduce spasticity and clonus; and decrease
inflammation and edema. The therapist should closely monitor the use of cold with patients, since cold
can cause skin burn. Cold can be transferred through
conduction and evaporation.

Conduction. This method of heat transfer occurs from
one object to another through physical contact.

• *Paraffin*: Paraffin is a mixture of seven parts paraffin
wax to one part mineral oil. The mixture is heated and
stored in a tub at 125–130° F. Paraffin is very useful
when the therapist is attempting to apply superficial
heat to an area that is hard to reach, such as the fingers of a patient who has rheumatoid arthritis.

  • **General Procedure**: Before the patient dips an
  extremity into paraffin, the patient should wash
  thoroughly to prevent contamination. The patient

then dips the hand into the tub 6–12 times, or as tolerated, while being sure to lift the hand completely out of the tub between dips. The therapist should then wrap the hand in a plastic bag and towel or other insulated fabric mitt/cover with the paraffin applied for 10–20 minutes. It is also good practice to elevate the patient's hand on an inclined surface, stack of towels, or pillow to help prevent edema. The patient should hold the hand still, since movement of the hand would break the paraffin seal and allow the heating benefit to escape.

- **Contraindications**: A patient who has open wounds should not apply paraffin. Paraffin is a type of heat that may cause vasodilation, so a patient with severe or moderate edema should also not use this modality. Other conditions that are contraindicated for paraffin treatment include fever, active bleeding, site of malignancy, peripheral vascular disease, and cardiac or arterial insufficiency. Caution should be used when applying heat to a patient who has Sensory deficits, slight Edema, or confusion.

- *Hot Packs*: Packs which contain silicate gel are heated and stored in a hydrocollator, or unit which contains water that is heated to 158°–176° F. The pack is generally able to retain heat for one-half hour.

  - **General Procedure**: Since the packs are heated to a level that can burn and cause tissue damage, hot packs are applied to the patient with towels or other insulated fabric pieces placed between the skin and the packs. Clothing and jewelry should be removed from the area being treated. Post, Lee, and Syen (1995) recommend 6–8 layers of fabric between the packs and the patient's skin. The therapist should check the patient's skin for redness or blotching after the packs have been applied for 5 minutes. If the patient complains of too much heat or the skin

Physical Agent Modalities (PAMs)

is red, more layers of insulation should be added between the packs and the skin. Treatment should last for 15–30 minutes. Hot packs may be applied to a patient who has open wounds.

- **Contraindications**: Heat is contraindicated with a patient who has moderate to severe edema, fever, active bleeding, site of malignancy, peripheral vascular disease, and cardiac and arterial insufficiency. Caution should be used when applying heat to a patient who has Sensory deficits, slight Edema, or confusion. This modality serves as an alternative to paraffin for the patient who has an open wound since hot packs may be used on open wounds unless otherwise indicated by the physician.

Convection. Heat transfer may occur through the motion of fluid surrounding tissues.

- *Hydrotherapy*: The physical properties of water can benefit affected body parts during immersion in many ways. Thermal effects occur similarly to the application of superficial thermal agents; however, the patient's body may respond systemically since more body surface is generally affected during hydrotherapy. Warm temperatures will initially increase blood pressure and heart rate, but vasodilation will occur and decrease blood pressure. Cold temperatures will cause vasoconstriction, which will increase blood pressure and decrease heart rate. Water creates buoyancy of the body near the surface of the water, which can assist the patient with movement. If body parts are immersed below the surface of the water, water creates resistance to movement for strengthening benefits. The density of water helps support the affected body part, which can decrease stress on the joints. The pressure of water helps promote circulation. Mechanical devices can agitate the water, which helps with wound debridement and pain relief.

- *Whirlpool* is the most common form of hydrotherapy. The various benefits of whirlpool treatment include debridement of wounds from water agitation, massage of the affected tissues, buoyancy and resistance of water against movement which can promote active movement and exercise during whirlpool.

  → *General Procedure*: When using whirlpool as a thermal modality, the water should be heated to 100°–105° F for upper limbs and 100°–102° F for lower limbs. If necessary, the water can be heated to 110° F, but full body immersion should occur in water which is 100° or below. Treatment may be completed for 10–20 minutes as tolerated by the patient. If using the whirlpool for wound care, a sterilizing agent must be added during treatment. Care should be taken to sanitize the whirlpool following every treatment.

  → *Contraindications*: See general hydrotherapy contraindications below.

- **Pool Therapy** may be used with patients for relaxation, increased circulation, increased motion, strengthening, stress reduction to joints, and leisure. Patients with the following diagnoses may benefit from aquatic therapy: mild spastic Cerebral palsy, orthopedic and musculoskeletal conditions, neurologic disorders, and rheumatoid arthritis. See Aquatic therapy for further discussion of treatment and specific contraindications.

- **Contrast Bath** is used to help decrease edema or Hypersensitivity. Patients with the following diagnoses may benefit from this modality: rheumatoid arthritis, joint sprains, muscle strains, reflex sympathetic dystrophy, or mild peripheral vascular diseases. See Edema for further discussion of treatment and specific contraindications.

- **General Contraindications of Hydrotherapy**: Hydrotherapy is contraindicated for patients with the following diagnoses/conditions: fever, infections, Sensory deficits, trauma or hemorrhage, sites of malignancy, bleeding disorders, cardiac instability, inability to communicate pain, atrophic skin, acute edema (except with contrast baths), ischemic areas, poor thermal regulation, and immature scar tissue.
- *Fluidotherapy*. A limb can be placed in a fluidotherapy machine which circulates finely ground corn husks in warm air (102°–118° F.). This heating mechanism has proven to be an excellent modality for raising the temperature of tissue in hands and feet. Benefits include heat as well as desensitization, massage, and slight resistance while providing an environment conducive to active motion/exercise.
  - **General Procedure**: The machine should be started prior to treatment, so that the particles are warm when treatment begins. The temperature ranges from 102°–125° F, and this should be set according to the patient's tolerance. The patient then places the limb in the machine, and the therapist should tightly fasten the band around the patient's limb to avoid particles from exiting the machine. Treatment lasts 20–30 minutes.
  - **Contraindications**: Patients who have open wounds or edema should not use fluidotherapy unless the wound is covered with a plastic bag. Care should be taken with patients who have Sensory deficits. See Paraffin or Hot packs above for general contraindications/precautions when using heat.

Conversion. The final method of heat transfer occurs when a modality creates internal friction to generate heat.
- *Ultrasound*: This machine produces sound waves, which can penetrate tissue to cause vibration of its molecules, resulting in heat from friction. Ultrasound

is helpful with the management of patients with the following diagnoses/conditions: scar tissue/keloids, tendinitis, bursitis, joint contractures, myositis ossificans, pain, and muscle spasm.

- **General Procedure**: A small instrument called a transducer applies sound waves through a gel is applied to the patient's skin for improved transmission to tissues. Ultrasound produces deep heat, which penetrates deeper than the previously mentioned modalities, usually to a depth of 1 cm. Sound waves can be set to cycle at a frequency of 1 MHz or 3 MHz. When cycling at 1 MHz, tissue is heated at a depth of 5 cm. Tissue can be heated more superficially at a depth of 3 cm if the therapist uses the 3-MHz setting. The strength of ultrasound is also set by programming the intensity of the sound waves, which are measured in watts per square centimeter. Intensity can range between .25–3.0 W/cm^2 during treatment; however, most treatment occurs between 1.0–2.0 W/cm.^{2} If applying ultrasound for thermal benefit, then *continuous wave* should be used. If mechanical benefit is the goal, then *pulsed wave* should be used. When placing the transducer on the patient's skin, small circular motions should be used to help avoid overheating a specific spot and the therapist should maintain even contact between the transducer with the treatment site. Also, the intensity of the waves should be reduced when using ultrasound over bony prominences. Once the ultrasound has been started, the head of the transducer should immediately applied to the patient's skin. Sound waves cannot be transmitted through air, so the crystal of the transducer may shatter or depolarize if not permitted to transmit its waves. Ultrasound is applied to the affected area for a duration of 8–10 minutes. A patient has this modality applied for 6–12 treatment sessions.

- Ultrasound may also be used as a nonthermal agent to help drive topical medication into deeper tissue, which is called Phonophoresis. The medications most commonly used include local anesthetics and corticosteroids. This modality may be 1 time a day for up to 10 days. The transducer may be set at a frequency of 1 or 2 Mhz and an intensity of 1–3 W/cm^2 for a duration of 5–7 minutes per site. Patients with the following diagnoses/conditions may benefit from phonophoresis: epicondylitis, tendinitis, tenosynovitis, bursitis, capsulitis, fasciitis, strains, contractures, osteoarthritis, impingement of shoulder, scar tissue, adhesions, and neuromas.
- **General Contraindications of Ultrasound**: Ultrasound should not be used over the following areas: heart, pacemakers, brain, eyes, laminectomized spine, testes, carotid sinus, cervical ganglia, acute joint pathologies, active bleeding, thrombophlebitic sites, growth plates, infected bone or other sites of infection, sites of malignancy, and fluid-filled cavities. Care should be taken to avoid overheating specific sites when using ultrasound over metal implants/hardware.

Cryotherapy. Cold is used in treatment to help decrease Edema, inflammation, and pain, as well as reduce spasticity and clonus. The application of cold results in vasoconstriction, the decrease of peripheral nerve conduction velocity, and increased stiffness due to decreased elasticity of tissue (Michlovitz, 1990b).

- *Cold Packs*: These silicone gel packs are stored in a freezer at 23°–45° F. When applied to a patient's skin, a moist towel should be placed between the pack and the patient's skin to prevent tissue damage. Cold packs should be applied for 15–30 minutes.
- *Ice Packs*: Plastic bags can be filled with ice and used for cooling if cold packs are not available. Ice packs

are actually colder on the skin than cold packs. The therapist again places a moist towel between the pack and the patient's skin. Ice packs should be applied for 10–20 minutes. After completing a home program, the patient can complete this cooling at home with ice in a plastic bag or a bag of frozen vegetables.

- *Ice Massage*: Water can be frozen in styrofoam, plastic, or paper cups. Following exercise, the therapist can retrieve a cup from the freezer, tear the bottom from the cup, and use the top half of the cup to hold the ice. The therapist should massage over the affected area for 5–10 minutes until the skin becomes numb.

- *Vapocoolant Sprays*: The most commonly used spray for superficial cooling is fluori-methane. The therapist should spray two or three times across an area of the skin where the patient complains of pain during stretch of a limb. Care should be taken so the skin is not frosted. After the skin has been sprayed, the therapist should stretch the limb and attempt to increase the ROM. This superficial cooling does not have the same stiffening effect as ice that is applied for a longer duration.

- *Cold Baths*: Body parts can also be immersed into a container filled with ice and water. The water temperature should range between 55°–65° F. The patient should place the affected part in the water 10–20 minutes, or as tolerated. If a patient is unable to tolerate the ice bath, the therapist can strain the ice out of the water immediately before the patient inserts his or her limb, which will allow the water to slightly heat back toward room temperature quicker.

- *General Contraindications of Cryotherapy*: Patients with the following diagnoses/conditions should not have cryotherapy applied: Raynaud's phenomenon, extreme hypersensitivity, compromised circulation, peripheral vascular disease, cardiac or respiratory involvement, initial stage of wound healing, an inability to communicate pain, severe hypertension, replantations, and crush injuries. Caution should be taken when applying cryotherapy to a patient who has Sensory deficits, as well as with the elderly or very young patient.

Electrical Modalities (Cummings, 1992; Kloth, 1992). Electrical current in small increments can help excite nerve or muscle tissue to help promote the restoration of lost function. The flow of electrons is able to transfer to the flow of ions within biological tissues through the application of electrodes to the patient's skin. The flow of ions in biological tissue is then able to produce an action potential within a nerve. Larger cutaneous nerves, which are closer to the surface of the skin, are the first nerves to be stimulated. A patient may report a "tingling" sensation, which results from the firing of the cutaneous nerves. If the amplitude is increased, the deeper motor nerves can be stimulated, resulting in muscle contraction. Research has shown that the application of electrical modalities can also increase local blood flow, stimulate soft tissue regeneration, increase levels of endorphins in the blood, and increase the absorption of fluid (Edema) from the affected site. The treatment of pain is also based on the gate-control theory, which posits that electrical current can close the gates that allow the pain impulses to reach the brain. Electrical modalities can help decrease pain, increase movement/strength, decrease edema, and reeducate muscles.

- *General Contraindications/Precautions to Electrotherapy*: Patients with the following diagnoses/conditions should not receive electrotherapy treatment: cardiac problems and/or pacemakers, active cancer/malignancy, local infections (except if use is for wound healing), decreased cutaneous sensation, pregnancy, seizure disorders, thrombotic blood vessels, fresh fractures, fusion, sutured nerves or tendons, eyes, edema, active hemorrhage, site of the carotid sinus, and on the anterior chest wall. Care should be taken when using electrical current with a patient who has high blood pressure, circulatory problems, peripheral vascular disease, problems communicating pain, or small body mass.

- **Iontophoresis**: This modality utilizes continuous low-voltage current that flows in one direction (DC current), otherwise known as galvanic current. Current of this type helps to promote wound and fracture healing. When ions are applied to the patient's skin, this current helps drive the ions into underlying tissue. This process is called iontophoresis. Different topical medications which contain ions can be applied to help facilitate various processes such as the following: reduce edema with corticosteroids, reduce pain with local anesthetics, relax muscle with magnesium sulfate, reduce calcium deposits with acetic acid, treat infections with copper sulfate, heal wounds with zinc oxide, or soften scars and adhesions with sodium chloride. Iontophoresis uses a current ranging from micoramperes up to 30 mA. One smaller active electrode is used with a larger dispersive electrode. The electrical unit should be set so that its polarity is the same as the medication being used. This will cause the current to repel the ions and drive them into the treatment site. The active electrode should be applied to the treatment site, while the dispersive electrode is applied ipsilaterally on the same general body area.
  - → *Contraindications*: Patients who have decreased sensation should not have DC current applied, since DC current can burn the skin. Patients should also not have medications applied, which cause the patient to have an allergic reaction.
- **Microcurrent Electrical Neuromuscular Stimulation (MENS)**: Use of low frequency and intensity

current so that the current is not sensed by the patient. This type of modality may be used to help reduce acute or chronic pain, reduce inflammation, reduce spasm, and promote healing of bones, nerves, or connective tissue. The efficacy of this modality is controversial.

- **Transcutaneous Electrical Nerve Stimulation (TENS)**: This modality helps decrease pain, based on the endorphin release principle and on the gate-control theory principle. Both acute and chronic pain may be relieved by TENS. The application of this device may help a patient who needs to begin movement following surgery, such as capsulotomy or Tenolysis, but complains of pain. TENS can be set at a short pulse duration, a frequency of 50–100 Hz, and an amplitude of 10–30mA (or within limits of perception). This setting brings relief that may last 1–3 hours within 1–20 minutes of application; however, relief may also end immediately following application. This setting is based on the gate control theory. TENS may also be set at a long pulse duration, a frequency of 1–4 Hz, and an amplitude of 30–80 mA (or until a slight motor response occurs). This setting brings relief within 20–30 minutes of application, but lasts from 2–6 hours following treatment. This setting is based on the endorphin release theory. When using conventional mode TENS (50–100 Hz), the electrodes may be placed at the local site of pain. If using low frequency TENS (1–4 Hz), the electrodes should be placed in the segmental myotome that is related to the involved area. Electrodes may also be placed on motor, trigger or acupuncture points (Gersh, 1992). Once educated, the patient can apply TENS daily as needed for pain.
- **Neuromuscular Electrical Stimulation (NMES)**: This modality helps reeducate and/or strengthen muscles, reduce atrophy, gain ROM, and reduce spasticity through the stimulation of antagonist muscles. NMES

uses an interrupted current to allow the muscle to relax between contractions. The electrodes should be placed on motor points of the muscles being stimulated, and the current should be increased until a response is demonstrated. If the therapist uses unipolar motor point stimulation, one electrode is small and the other large. The same amount of current passes through both electrodes; however, the current is more dense in the small electrode. The small electrode is the active one and should be placed on the motor point. When finding the motor point, refer to a motor point chart if possible. If no references are available, the motor point tends to be in the middle of the muscle belly. Lightly place the active electrode on the approximate motor point. While the unit delivers current, slowly slide the active electrode around on the skin until the strongest contraction is demonstrated. The active electrode can then be firmly attached to the motor point site. The larger, dispersive electrode is often placed distally over the tendinous portion of the muscle. Unipolar stimulation may be applied to a patient with peripheral nerve injury or tendon transplant. Bipolar stimulation utilizes two equally-sized electrodes with equal strength of current. The electrodes may both be placed on the muscle being stimulated; however, the distance between the electrodes should at least be the length of diameter of one electrode to prevent short-circuiting. The unit can produce a contraction near a frequency of 30 pps. A ratio of 1 unit of "on time" to 5 units of "off time" is a good starting point if using NMES with a patient who has hemiplegia. Orthopedic patients benefit from a 1:3 ratio, while a patient who needs to increase muscle strength will benefit from a 1:1 ratio of "on time" to "off time." The electrical unit should always be turned back to zero following treatment. Duration of treatment can range between 10–45 minutes, depending on the goal of treatment and the patient's tolerance. NMES can also be referred to functional electrical stimulation (FES) if applied while asking the patient to complete functional activities.

- **High-Voltage Galvanic Stimulation (HVGS)**: This modality may also be referred to as high voltage pulsed current (HVPC). It is used to treat pain and edema, improve circulation, reeducate muscles, reduce muscle guarding, decrease atrophy/increase strength, or heal wounds. The active electrode should be placed over the involved site, while the dispersive electrode is placed on the body at a good distance from the treatment site. Some dispersive electrodes are so large that they must be placed on the back or abdomen. This electrical unit differs from low voltage units in that the current has a higher voltage (up to 500 volts) and waves that are unidirectional and close together. This modality may treat various conditions using different settings. Please refer to a specific HVGS treatment table for settings and treatment time (e.g., Hayes, 1984).

- **Interferential Electrical Stimulation**: This modality is sometimes referred to as interference current (IFC). It is used to treat chronic pain and edema. The electrical unit has two equal currents delivered to the affected tissue at two different frequencies. This causes a summation of current (70–100 mA) which is greater than the current provided to the tissue by TENS, and this current is then able to stimulate both sensory and motor nerve fibers. Stimulation results in muscle contraction of deeper, larger muscles, which may be pain-relieving. The IFC electrical unit may be set at the maximal output which the patient is able to tolerate.

Pinch.   Usually referred to when testing a patient's finger strength. A pinch meter is used for measuring a patient's palmar, lateral, and tip pinch in pounds of pressure. See <u>Prehension</u>.

PIP.   Proximal interphalangeal.

Place and Hold.   Activities completed with the therapist's assistance by persons who demonstrate weakness or the inability to control movement. The therapist assists the patient with movement, such as flexing the shoulder to 90°, and then asks the patient to attempt to hold the extremity in that position. The therapist should decrease the amount of assistance being given to hold the affected extremity in place, but not withdraw assistance completely at the beginning of place and hold activities. As the patient increases voluntary muscle contraction, the therapist should decrease assistance until the patient is able to both place and hold the extremity in the desired position independently. See Motor control problems.

Placing Reaction or Placing Reflex.   See Reflexes and reactions.

Plantar Flexion.   A joint motion at the ankle which results in the toes being pulled downward away from the knee. This is ankle joint flexion, which is often mislabeled as extension. See Appendix E for the normal range of this motion.

Plantar Grasp Reflex.   See Reflexes and reactions.

Poetry Therapy.   Use of poetry to help clients to express their feelings and innermost thoughts. The poetry is designed to convey a vivid and imaginative sense of experience. It can be insightful in discovering a person's fantasies, desires, and fears.

Pool Therapy.   A physical agent modality which can be classified as hydrotherapy. See Aquatic therapy for specifics of treatment and further discussion.

Position in Space.   The ability to understand terms which define position such as over, under, above, beneath, and so on, and then apply those to objects. See Cognitive-perceptual deficits for further discussion and treatment.

Positioning.   Patients who are unable to move themselves or particular body parts must be positioned appropriately by the therapist. Incorrect positioning can result in contractures, foot drop, subluxation, decubitus ulcers, pain, disfigurement, and decreased functional ability. A patient must be positioned correctly while in bed as well as while in a wheelchair or dining room chair. Often, common items such as pillows can be used to promote proper alignment; however, special equipment should be fabricated or ordered as needed.

Bed Positioning

- Positioning for patients with hemiplegia, according to neurodevelopmental treatment by Bobath (1978).
- This is the preferred position for patients who have hemiplegia. Lying on the affected side helps provide input through weightbearing. The patient should be positioned with the head symmetrical; a pillow may be used if the head is not flexed too much. Next, the affected arm should be fully protracted and flexed at the shoulder to at least 90° with the elbow flexed and the forearm supinated so that the affected hand is under the pillow. The elbow may also be extended with the wrist slightly off the bed to help encourage wrist extension. The affected leg should be extended at the hip and slightly flexed at the knee, while the unaffected leg is supporting on a pillow in hip and knee flexion for comfort.
- Lying on the nonaffected side begins with the head positioned symmetrically on a pillow. Again, the affected shoulder is fully protracted and flexed to 90°. The affected arm should be supported on a pillow so that the wrist is placed in neutral and not allowed to flex. The affected leg should also be supported by a pillow so that the hip and knee are flexed and the foot and ankle are supported so that the foot does not invert.
- Lying supine begins with the head symmetrical. A pillow should be placed under the affected shoulder so that it is

symmetrical with the nonaffected shoulder; however, care should be taken so that it is not overly raised as this could result in anterior subluxation. The affected arm should be slightly flexed and abducted at the shoulder, extended at the elbow, and supinated or neutral at the forearm with the hand open and a pillow supporting the entire arm.

- If a patient has sustained a brain injury, sidelying is the preferred position. The supine position may facilitate the Tonic labyrinthine reflex, which will govern the patient's position. The patient may lay on either side with a small pillow to support the head in alignment with the trunk. Both upper extremities should be protracted at the shoulders in slight shoulder flexion. A pillow may be placed between the arms to prevent horizontal adduction of the uppermost arm. The patient's wrists should be extended and cones may be placed in the patient's hands to prevent contractures due to increased tone. The lower extremities should be slightly flexed at the knee and hip with a pillow to prevent hip adduction and internal rotation of the uppermost leg. Pillows may also be needed behind the patient's back to help the patient maintain a sidelying position. Padded boots may be applied to the feet to prevent pressure areas on the feet and to position the ankle near 90° flexion to prevent foot drop. If the patient does lay in supine, pillows should be used to protract the shoulders. The upper extremities should be abducted slightly and externally rotated. Cones may also be used in this position if a patient demonstrates increased tone.

Wheelchair Positioning

- The first step of positioning is to produce correct placement and position of the patient's pelvis. The patient should be sitting on the pelvis symmetrically rather than having more weight on one hip than the other. A wedge cushion may be used to support the side of the pelvis that is supporting more weight in order to redistribute the patient's weight equally.

- The patient's pelvis should be in neutral or slightly tilted anteriorly. A solid seat may need to be installed since a regular fabric seat encourages posterior pelvic tilt, which will lead to poor posture, as well as internal rotation and adduction of the hips. A small lumbar roll also facilitates anterior pelvic tilt.

- When sitting, the patient should have the hips at 90° flexion. A wedge cushion can be used with the higher side of the wedge placed toward the front of the wheelchair seat, at the patient's knees, to achieve proper hip position.

- A seat belt provides safety as well as good positioning. The belt should fasten along the lower pelvis area to help continue proper pelvic tilt and even weightbearing through the hips.

- Pads may be placed along the lateral aspect of the thighs to prevent the patient from excessively abducting the hips.

- A pad or swing-away abductor may be placed between the patient's thighs to prevent the patient from excessively adducting the hips. An abductor that can be lowered under the chair as needed preserves the patient's ability to transfer, while a pad that is permanently in the chair can increase the assistance needed for the patient to transfer.

- If a patient tends to slide forward in the wheelchair, the above abductor or wedge cushion may be indicated. A larger wedge cushion, called an antithrust cushion, may be used to prevent the patient from falling out of the chair. This cushion may cause hip flexion greater than 90°; however, if the patient's is at risk of hurting him or herself by falling, the cushion should be used.

- If the patient is prone to skin breakdown from poor nutrition or incontinence, a gel cushion or other pressure-relieving device should be used in the seat. Patients with spinal cord injury are specifically at risk due to absent or decreased sensation and decreased ability to reposition oneself.

- The patient's trunk should be aligned with the pelvis. A solid seat back may be required to prevent the patient from leaning back too far into the existing fabric seat back. This back may be reclined 10°–15° to align the trunk and head with the pelvis. If trunk flexion is an extreme problem, the seat may be reclined farther to prevent the patient from falling out of the wheelchair. Care should be taken during meals to return the patient to a more upright position for safety in swallowing.

- If the patient tends to lean to one side, lateral supports may be used to elongate the shortened side of the trunk.

- A patient may have shoulder straps applied to the wheelchair to prevent falls from extreme trunk flexion. This may be viewed as a restraint, so the proper channels should be used to approve this positioning device.

- The patient's knees and ankles should be flexed as close to 90° as possible. The patient's feet should be placed against the footrests in neutral with the entire foot supported; pronation/supination and inversion/eversion should be avoided at the ankle. Calf pads or straps behind the footrests can be used to help the patient keep the feet on the footrests. Guards can be placed along the front of the footrests to prevent the patient from extending the feet over the front edge of the footrest.

- The ideal upper extremity position is as follows: neutral scapular elevation/depression with slight protraction; slight shoulder flexion, abduction, and external rotation; comfortable elbow flexion supported by the arm rests; forearm pronation; neutral wrist flexion/extension and ulnar/radial deviation; comfortable slight finger flexion; and thumb abduction. If the patient has hemiplegia or weakness, the affected arm should be supported to prevent Subluxation. A lapboard may be used across the armrests of the wheelchair both as support for the upper extremities and as a surface for completing activities such as feeding or exercises. A special arm trough may be purchased or fabricated to prevent the affected arm from sliding off of the armrest. An inclined cushion may be used if the patient demonstrates Edema. If the patient demonstrates flaccid or spastic hemiplegia, the affected hand may require a Splint to prevent contractures and maintain skin integrity. See Splints, CVA, and Edema for more specific instructions concerning these conditions.

- The patient's head should be aligned with the trunk for safety in swallowing. The neck should be extended so that the head is upright with the chin slightly tucked. If the patient is not able to hold the head upright, a head rest may be used to support the head from the back, side or front. If a front support is needed during eating, it is beneficial if this device is detachable to make transfers easier.

Positive Supporting Reaction. See Reflexes and reactions.

Positive Symptoms. In a psychiatric illness such as Schizophrenia, positive symptoms represent an excess or distortion of normal functions, for example, normal suspicion becomes delusional thinking or illusions become hallucinations. Other examples of positive symptoms include disorganized speech and thinking, bizarre dressing, and exaggerated postures or hand movements.

Post-Polio Syndrome. A disorder resulting in progressive weakness that may be accompanied by fatigue, pain, cold intolerance, and breathing difficulties. This disorder occurs in persons who had poliomyelitis in the past, and the cause of the recurrence of symptoms of polio may be linked to overuse or disuse of muscles as well as motor unit dysfunction.

Specific Treatments

- Complete aerobic exercise for strengthening, but avoid fatigue and pain
- Train the patient to use a new orthosis or power wheelchair if applicable
- Teach the patient energy conservation and work simplification techniques
- Assist the patient with establishing a diet to help lose weight and increase the patient's energy level
- Establish a time management program that alternates periods of activity with periods of rest
- Instruct the patient on Stress management and relaxation techniques
- Encourage the patient to join a support group for socialization and adjustment to the disease
- Provide education on assistive devices and equipment that can increase or maintain the patient's independence with Self-care activities
- Modify work or leisure tasks as needed to allow the patient to continue with previous responsibilities/tasks

Contraindications/Precautions

- Avoid overexertion and fatigue since this could result in a loss of muscle strength for a duration of days

Postrotary Nystagmus (PRN). A normal reaction of the eyes in reaction to the body being rotated in a swing. The eyeballs respond by constantly moving in a cyclical direction. PRN is assessed by therapists using sensory integrative therapy.

Post-traumatic Stress Disorder. An anxiety disorder that occurs in response to a traumatic event such as a war time experience, natural disaster, airplane crash, parental abuse, or physical/mental torture. The symptoms include recurring vivid memories of the past experience causing insomnia, recurrent nightmares, hypervigilance, and other symptoms related to Anxiety. The disorder can last for

Post-traumatic Stress Disorder. *(continued)*
many years. <u>Stress management</u> techniques, relaxation
therapies and expressive media can be effective in helping
the client.

Postural Alignment.   The coordination and integration
of joints during movements to maintain neutral positions;
for example, in the wrist, elbow, shoulder, torso, and hip.
When teaching correct biomechanical principles in standing, sitting, lifting, and transferring objects, consider postural alignment.

Posterior.   See <u>Anatomical position</u>.

Postural Control.   The ability to use righting and equilibrium adjustments to maintain balance during functional
movements such as returning to an upright position after
bending down, prolonged standing in an awkward position
such as in a job, or dancing. <u>Tai chi</u>, <u>Yoga</u>, and <u>Range of
motion</u> dance can be modified to meet the individual's
needs for improving postural control.

Posterior.   See <u>Anatomical positions</u>.

Postural tone.   The amount of <u>Muscle tone</u> necessary in
the trunk muscles that is great enough to allow a person to
remain upright against the force of gravity, but low enough
to permit movement such as bending, <u>Righting</u>, or <u>Equilib-
rium reactions</u>.

Prader-Willi Syndrome.   A congenital condition that
results in <u>Mental retardation</u>, short stature, inability of sexual organs to mature properly, and obesity.

Praxis.   Ability to conceive and execute a motor act such as
dressing, brushing one's teeth or driving a car. The motor
act is carried out in a sequential pattern of purposeful movements. A task analysis can be useful in analyzing a motor
activity into discrete actions, such as tying shoelaces. Individuals with brain damage such as in cerebrovascular acci-

dents can develop <u>Apraxia</u>. This skill may also be referred to as motor planning. A patient who is not able to brush his or her hair even though the patient's motor, sensory, and coordination abilities are intact demonstrates apraxia. See <u>Cognitive-perceptual deficits</u> for treatment and further discussion.

Preferred Provider Organizations (PPOs). Networks of health care professionals who provide services to a group health plan such as an <u>HMO</u>. PPOs are paid a capitation fee for each subscriber to the plan and on that basis they provide comprehensive health care services.

Prehension. The act of bringing the thumb and fingers into contact in order to manipulate small objects.

Types of Prehension

- *Palmar Prehension*: Also referred to as the three-jaw chuck pinch, this pattern combines opposition and rotation of the thumb with flexion of the index and long fingers for pad-to-pad contact of the fingers and thumb. This pattern is used when tying shoelaces or picking small objects up off of a flat surface.
- *Lateral Prehension*: This prehension pattern is comprised of opposition of the thumb to the radial side of the index finger (either the middle or distal phalanx). This pattern is used when turning a key or holding a fork.
- *Tip Prehension*: This pattern combines opposition and flexion of the IP joint of the thumb with PIP and DIP flexion of the index finger so that the tips of the distal phalanxes are touching. This pattern is used when picking up a very small object such as a hair pin or penny.

Prescriptive Exercise. Any physical activity that is planned, purposeful, and structured. It includes aerobic and anaerobic exercises, isometric, isotonic, stretching, relaxation, and passive motions. In general exercise is beneficial for almost every client. It is used to meet the health needs of every individual. As part of an occupational therapy pro-

Prescriptive Exercise. *(continued)*

gram, prescriptive exercise is goal directed, meaningful to the client and provides sensorimotor, cognitive and psychosocial stimulation (Wykoff, 1993). In designing a therapeutic exercise program for an individual the therapist should consider the (a) type of exercise, such as walking, swimming, progressive relaxation; (b) duration of time in doing the exercise; (c) intensity of the exercise, such as mild, moderate or intense; (d) frequency such as daily, 2–3 times a week or weekly; and (e) methods to increase compliance to exercise schedule, such as daily monitoring and external reinforcement. To be successful the therapist should consider the following:

- Select an exercise that is meaningful to the client.
- Incorporate the exercise into the client's everyday schedule.
- As a general target goal have the client engage in moderate exercise for 30 to 35 minutes daily.
- Have the client keep a diary of exercise.
- Encourage the client to evaluate the effects of the exercise.
- Have the client incorporate an aerobic, relaxation and stretching exercise in the morning or early evening.

Pressure. A technique that can be used for either facilitation or inhibition of Muscle tone. If facilitating tone, the pressure is applied with the thumb, first, and second digits placed in close proximity to one another, while the therapist begins a stretch of the muscle fibers of a muscle belly. The stimulus should be applied for 3 seconds. As the Stretch occurs, the thumb will gradually move away from the first and second digits. Lotion may need to be applied to prevent heat friction. If inhibiting tone, the pressure is applied to the tendinous insertion of the muscle being inhibited. For example, if inhibiting the biceps, then deep pressure should be applied to the inside of the elbow or the bicipital aponeurosis. A hard surface helps inhibit tone to a greater extent, which explains the technique of placing a cone in a patient's hand or fabricating a hard Splint. See

Motor control problems, Rood approach for further discussion of inhibition techniques.

Prevocational Evaluation. Program to assess a client's ability to work, for example, in a sheltered workshop, competitive employment, or as homemaker.

Primary Prevention. Prevention of the initial onset of a disease, for example, the prevention of polio with a vaccination.

Prime Mover. A muscle or group of muscles primarily responsible for a particular movement. For example, the prime movers for elbow flexion are the biceps, brachialis, and brachioradialis.

Problem Solving. Cognitive ability that entails recognizing and defining a problem, identifying alternative solutions, selecting the most feasible solution, devising a plan to implement solution, evaluating the outcome, and readjusting the solution. Problem solving is an important task of the occupational therapist such as in Ergonomics where the therapist devises a plan to prevent injury on the job, Home health where the therapist helps the client to be independent in Self-care activities, and in Psychosocial rehabilitation where the client learns how to Self-regulate stress. Problem solving by the client is encouraged through trial-and-error learning.

Problem-Oriented Medical Record (POMR). Systematic method of recording progress notes in a patient's chart that prioritizes the symptoms and problems and includes a plan to treat these problems. The initial notes are periodically evaluated and progress notes are recorded. SOAP notes are part of a problem-oriented record.

Problem Solving. Ability to apply current knowledge to create solutions when new problems or situations arise. This is a cognitive function that should be tested following brain injury or in the presence of disease processes that can

Problem Solving. *(continued)*
alter brain activity. See <u>Cognitive-perceptual deficits</u> for further discussion and treatment.

Procrustean Bed. Applying a treatment method such as a panacea to all patients regardless of individual differences and needs. For example, applying a treatment procedure to all patients with arthritis, as well as to all patients with cancer, without regard to the individual and specific needs of each patient. In this method, the patient is fitted to the treatment method rather than, in good treatment, being given the best and most effective treatment method.

Prodromal. The initial symptoms that can lead to precipitating an episode of a disease in a vulnerable individual.

Professional Standard Review Organization (PSROs). Founded by the U.S. Congress in 1972 to ensure that health care services provided under Medicare, Medicaid, or Maternal and Child Health programs were of acceptable professional quality.

Prognosis. Clinical forecast of the probable course of the illness and the eventual outcome of the disease or condition. For example, the prognosis of an individual diagnosed with <u>Schizophrenia</u> will depend on the age of the initial onset, the severity of symptoms, intelligence level, and environmental factors.

Progressive Relaxation. A treatment method developed by Edmund Jacobson (1929, 1978) based on systematically tensing and relaxing muscle groups in the body. The procedure involves identifying a local state of tension and relaxing it away by learning to control all of the skeletal musculature through systematic muscle tension and relaxation. In practicing progressive relaxation the client should consider:
- Set aside a specific time during the day such as before dinner and about 15 to 20 minutes to practice.
- Block out distracting noises or interruptions.

- Use a firm mattress, tatami, or exercise mat.
- Have the client learn how to flex and relax individual muscles starting with the upper extremities, head and neck, and then lower extremities.
- Incorporate relaxing music into the exercise.
- As a precaution do not move muscles that are tender, strained or produce pain. The purpose of the exercise is to gently move flex and relax muscles in a progressive manner.
- Continuously have the client evaluate the benefits of the exercise.

PROM. See Passive range of motion.

Pronation. See Anatomical position.

Prone. A term which refers to the position of a patient while the patient lies on a horizontal surface with the stomach and front of the legs touching the supporting surface.

Proprioception. The ability to identify where body parts are in space. This is one of many components included in a sensory evaluation to test for deficits. See Sensory deficits for further discussion and treatment.

Proprioceptive Neuromuscular Facilitation. A traditional approach to the treatment of persons with motor control problems, specifically patients who have Parkinson's disease, spinal cord injury, arthritis, stroke, head injury, and Hand injuries. This approach is based on overall muscle movement patterns rather than individual muscle contractions. Other important principles include: normal development proceeds in a cervicocaudal and proximodistal direction, a person's nervous system can recall reflexes to help achieve movement, and the patient must practice for motor learning to occur (Kabat, H. 1961; Voss, 1967; Voss, Iota, & Myers, 1985).

Proprioceptive Sensation. Receiving and interpreting stimuli originating primarily in the joints and muscles, which gives us information about the position of bodily

Proprioceptive Sensation. *(continued)*
parts in space and in relation to each other; for example, touching the nose with a forefinger with eyes closed.

Prosthesis.   A device fabricated to substitute for a missing part of the body. Patients who have had parts of the body amputated may require a simple prosthesis for cosmetic reasons or a very complex electrically powered prosthesis for completing work tasks. See Amputation for further discussion and treatment.

Protective Arm Extension.   See Reflexes and reactions.

Protective Reaction.   A reaction of the extremities during an Equilibrium reaction. If equilibrium cannot be reestablished by the body, then the extremities will automatically abduct and/or extend to protect the body when falling. See Reflexes and reactions for further discussion.

Proximal.   See Anatomical position.

Proximal Traction Response.   Flexion of *all* flexor muscles of the upper extremity in response to a stretch of the flexor muscles at one joint of the upper extremity. For example, if the elbow flexors are stretched, then all muscles of that extremity will flex, resulting in a flexor synergy. See Motor control problems, Movement therapy of Brunnstrom.

Psychedelic.   A term popularized in the 1960s during the "hippie era" that referred to an altered state of consciousness and visual hallucinations produced by drugs such as mescaline, psilocybin, or lysergic acid diethylamide (LSD).

Psychiatric Diagnostic Interview.   An exploration of the patient's symptoms and problems; past psychiatric treatments, hospitalizations, and medications; medical history of past diseases, allergies, and bodily injuries; family history of mental illness; psychosocial development, education, occupation, family relationship, friendships, and sexual experiences; mental status examination: assessment of appearance, behavior, current mood, cognition, suicidal or homicidal thoughts, and reality testing.

Psychiatric Rehabilitation. Multidisciplinary approach with the goal of restoring function in social skills, self-care, leisure, and work (Anthony, 1979). Psychiatric rehabilitation refers to restoring function in an individual with a psychiatric disability.

Psychoanalysis. A systematic method of Psychotherapy founded by Sigmund Freud that employs free association, dream analysis, analyses of transference, and other psychodynamic techniques to help an individual understand the unconscious feelings and desires that shape his or her personality and behavior.

Psychodrama. A form of group Psychotherapy in which patients act out assigned roles. The therapeutic goals are to reduce emotional symptoms and encourage personal growth. The psychodrama includes a protagonist who is the center of the drama, alter egos who help the protagonist to think through identified issues, a director who sets the stage and scenes, and an audience who comment on the actions and give insight to the protagonist.

Psychodynamic. Refers to the understanding of the conscious and unconscious forces that motivate behavior, cause symptoms, and shape one's personality. Psychotherapists such as psychoanalysts use a psychodynamic approach in treating individuals with mental disorders.

Psychoeducational. In this approach, the therapist uses educational technology such as lecture, discussion, seminars, handouts, Role playing and video tapes in teaching clients how to deal more effectively with their illness. For example the therapist using a Group therapy format can help clients with arthritis to learn energy conservation methods, ergonomics, mechanics of lifting and methods to

Psychoeducational. (*continued*)

reduce stress. This approach has been effective with clients with depression, low back pain and stroke. The therapist designs the group by

- developing specific objectives for the clients such as, learn relaxation techniques
- organizing a time schedule for group such as, nine sessions once a week for one hour
- identifying course content, such as, demonstrating and practice with heart rate <u>Biofeedback</u> to increase relaxation or film on nutrition
- setting up homework assignments for clients to practice skills or exercise program
- having client keep diary of symptoms and progress of improvement
- having closure activity and follow-up recommendations.

Psychomotor agitation.   Describes the state of a client who is in constant motion with severe restlessness, pacing, wringing of hands, and purposeless activity accompanied by a high level of anxiety.

Psychoneuroimmunology.   Study of the relationships and interactions between the mind, central nervous system, autonomic nervous system, and endocrine system. It represents the effects of psychological states on the immune system. It has been found in some studies that extreme stress reactions can dampen the immune system and leave the individual vulnerable to disease.

Psychopathic.   Antisocial behavior such as violence, criminal activity, physical or sexual abuse, or related behaviors that reflect a lack of moral and ethical standards. Synonymous terms are sociopathic and antisocial reaction.

Psychosis.   A severe mental disorder characterized by delusions, hallucinations, thinking disturbances, and inability to perform activities of daily living as occurs in <u>Schizophrenia</u>, extreme <u>Depression</u>, dementia, and chronic alcoholism.

Psychosocial Skills and Psychological Components. The individual's abilities and characteristics to engage and interact in society and to express and control emotions. These include psychological Values, Interests, and Self-concept; social Role Performance, Conduct, Interpersonal skills, Self-expression, and management of Coping skills, Temporal planning, and Self-control.

Psychosomatic medicine. The study of the relationship of psychological factors and the etiology of physical and psychiatric disorders. Current investigators in psychosomatic medicine examine both the physical and psychological factors as causes and effects and treat mind and body as one.

Psychotherapy. Method of treating individuals with mental illnesses through verbal means. It originated from Sigmund Freud's work on Psychoanalysis and was called the "talking cure." The various schools of psychotherapy include Psychoanalytic, Client-centered, Rational-emotive, Cognitive, Cognitive-behavioral, Adlerian, Jungian, Behavior modification, Transactional analysis, and Psychodrama. Within these models there are many more frames of references in psychotherapy. As a treatment technique it relies primarily on the verbal interactions between the therapist and client. The methods used in psychotherapy vary considerably depending on the theoretical model espoused by the therapist. In general the phases in psychotherapy include

- establishing rapport and a therapeutic alliance with the client
- understanding the client's problems and making a tentative diagnosis
- helping the client to understand and gain insight into the causes of his or her problems
- setting goals for treatment that are mutually acceptable by therapist and client

- implementing treatment where the client learns and tests out new behaviors
- closure and discharge of the client.

Ptosis.   A condition in which the upper eyelid droops.

Quadriplegia.   Paralysis of all four extremities.

Quadruped.   The position referred to by Rood when a patient is bearing weight on all four extremities with shoulders flexed with elbows extended, and hips and knees flexed. See <u>Motor control problems</u>, <u>Rood</u> for further discussion and treatment.

Quality Assurance.   A system to measure the effectiveness of a hospital or treatment facility to meet standards of care established by governmental agencies or hospital associations. A quality assurance program in a hospital includes an evaluation component to identify problems and an action component to improve patient care.

Quality of Life.   Concept that implies that individuals have the capacity to determine what brings them most happiness in their lives. Factors such as being with one's family, being in one's home, ability to travel independently, food choices, expressing oneself through music and art, socializing with friends, and working at an interesting job are components of quality of life.

Ramiste's Phenomenon. A term used for a specific associated reaction when resistance against hip abduction or adduction in the noninvolved lower extremity elicits the same motion in the involved extremity. See <u>Motor control problems</u>, <u>Movement therapy of Brunnstrom</u>.

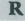

Range of Motion (Palmer & Epler, 1998). The amount of movement available at a joint, usually abbreviated ROM. A patient must have a functional range of motion in order to complete most functional activities; therefore, ROM may be included in a patient's plan of treatment as an adjunctive treatment to help increase the patient's independence with daily activities. The therapist should measure ROM if a patient demonstrates impairment to help monitor and document progress during treatment. The therapist uses a goniometer to measure the number of degrees available at a joint.

Methods of Measurement

- When measuring the range of most joints, the 180° system is used. The starting point of the joint motion (which begins from anatomical position) is 0° and the degrees increase toward 180° as the motion continues. When documenting measurements, the degrees for extension and flexion are written together as a range. If using the neutral zero method when measuring an impaired joint, then the number of degrees for the joint range are written as "extension limitation: 15° to 140°" or "flexion limitation: 0° to 100°." If hyperextension occurs at the joint, past the expected starting point, then that range is written separately as "hyperextension: 0° to 20°."

- Many therapists document the limitations using a different method. An impairment in extension is measured as the number of degrees the joint lacks from the starting position, or as "−15°". *Flexion* is written as the number of degrees from the starting position, or "100°." *Hyperextension* is measured as the number of degrees the joint has in addition to the normal range, or "+20°." So a patient who is able to hyperextend at the MCPs may

246

receive a range of "+20° to 90°," which denotes the range's starting and ending points. A therapist should check his or her facility's requirements for documenting ROM as methods can vary. Motion can be measured during active movement through the range, or while the therapist passively moves the joint through range. When possible, the therapist should compare limited ROM in a joint to the corresponding joint of the unaffected extremity. If this is not possible, the therapist should refer to a table of average ranges, which can be found in Appendix E.

Types

- **Active Range of Motion**: The amount of movement at a joint when the patient actively contracts appropriate muscles acting on that joint. The abbreviation commonly used is AROM. When possible, the therapist should compare limited ROM in a joint to the corresponding joint of the unaffected extremity. If this is not possible, the therapist should refer to a table of average ranges, which can be found in Appendix E.

- **Passive Range of Motion**: The amount of movement at a joint when the joint is moved through its range by an outside force, rather than by the muscles which act on that joint. The abbreviation commonly used is PROM. A therapist often passively moves body parts through range to help prevent stiffness and contractures when the muscles are too weak.

General Procedures for Testing

- The patient is seated comfortably. The joint to be measured is exposed so that bony landmarks and muscle contraction can be observed.

- The therapist should passively move the joint through its range to estimate the available ROM. The joint should be returned to its starting position.

- The therapist should place the goniometer with the stationary arm on the stationary part of the joint and the movable arm on the moving part. Bony landmarks should be identified and used to help find proper placement for the axis. The joint should be measured at the starting position, and the goniometer should then be removed from the joint. The patient should actively move the joint as far as possible toward the ending point of motion, or the therapist should passively move the joint through its range, without force, toward the ending point. The goniometer should be placed again and the joint should be measured at the ending position.

- If the patient is unable to reach the estimated ROM (PROM), then muscle weakness is limiting AROM. If AROM = PROM, but PROM is not equal to the unaffected extremity or average ranges, then joint limitation exists and PROM should also be measured. In the interest of time, if limitations in PROM are observed during the beginning estimation of ROM (prior to AROM), measurements for PROM can be taken at that time. If PROM or AROM are comparable from one arm to the other or to average ranges, then ROM can be recorded "within normal limits," and measurements do not need to be taken.

Functional ROM Testing. The therapist may use this abbreviated version of testing to screen the patient. If the patient demonstrates deficits, then the entire test should be given.

Procedure. The patient should be seated upright while the therapist asks the patient to complete the following motions. The therapist may demonstrate the motions if needed.

- *Trunk Flexion/Extension*: "Please reach down to your toes and then come back up."
- *Trunk Lateral Flexion*: "Please reach down to the floor to the left side of your chair with your left hand, and to the right side of your chair with your right hand."
- *Shoulder Flexion*: "Raise your arms up in front of you as high as you can."
- *Shoulder External Rotation*: "Place your hands behind your head or neck."

- *Shoulder Internal Rotation*: "Place your hands behind your back."
- *Shoulder Abduction*: "Raise your arms up and out to the side of you as high as you can."
- *Supination/Pronation*: "Turn your palms up toward the ceiling and then down toward the floor."
- *Elbow Flexion/Extension*: "Bend your elbows to touch your shoulders and then straighten them."
- *Wrist Flexion/Extension*: "Bend your wrist up and down."
- *Radial/Ulnar Deviation*: "Bend your hands out toward your small finger and then in toward your thumb."
- *Finger Flexion/Extension*: "Make a tight fist with each hand and then straighten your fingers."
- *Thumb Opposition*: "Touch the tip of each finger to the tip of your thumb."

The therapist should use this abbreviated test only if he or she knows and understands the full AROM test.

Contraindications

- Joint motion should *not* be measured or completed in the presence of the following conditions: myositis ossificans, joint dislocation, surgery or repair to any soft tissue surrounding the joint, or fractures which are not completely healed.
- Precautions should be used if the patient has osteoporosis, a Subluxation, inflammation at the joint, joint laxity, hemophilia, hematoma, or takes muscle relaxants or pain medication.
- When the therapist is unable to compare to the noninvolved extremity, refer to Appendix E, for average ranges of motion.

Treatment Methods

- **Active Assistive Range of Motion**. This technique is used when a patient does not have enough muscle strength to move a joint through its available range of motion. The therapist should hold the affected extremity

Range of Motion

near the joint being moved, with one hand stabilizing the joint and the other holding the moving part. As the patient actively attempts to move the body part, the therapist should only assist when needed. This technique is also referred to as Active-assisted range of motion, and the abbreviation listed in the patient's chart is A/AROM.

- Range of motion arc (the patient slides rings up and over a large arc)
- Bean bag activities: the patient slides the bags off a large table to either side or forward, or tosses the bags into a bucket placed at a distance
- Clothespins: the patient places clothespins as high as possible onto a vertical rod which is taller than the patient's highest reach
- ROM exercises/dowel or broomstick exercises: the patient can complete motions unassisted and actively, or the patient can use a dowel, broomstick, or towel to allow the unaffected extremity to assist the affected extremity through increased range
- Stacking cones or any bilateral clasped hands activity
- Reaching for items above the head
- Playing catch
- Washing tables with a wet rag
- Wiping vertical surfaces such as mirrors or walls
- Skateboard: the patient places the affected upper extremity on a skateboard to go from one side to the other or forward and back on the surface of a table
- Pulleys: the unaffected upper extremity can assist the affected upper extremity in reaching full shoulder flexion; in the same manner, the upper extremity bicycle allows the unaffected upper extremity to assist the affected upper extremity with elbow flexion and extension
- Ring tree: the patient may use one or both extremities to retrieve one ring at a time from a horizontal rod on one side of the "tree" and move it to a horizontal rod on the other side of the "tree"

- Finger ladder: the patient uses the fingers to inch up a small ladder on the wall (or can simply walk against the surface of the wall) to help assist shoulder flexion
- Balloon volleyball
- Large tabletop board games like giant checkers
- ROM dance program

Range of Motion Dance (ROM dance). A movement therapy comprised of expressive dance and relaxation techniques. It incorporates joint motion in all ranges to help individuals with joint and muscle limitations. It is also an educational process that assists individuals in improving their movement functioning through hands-on repatterning and verbal instruction.

Rational-Emotive Therapy (RET). A direct Psychotherapy technique originated by Albert Ellis (Ellis & Whiteley, 1979) that helps the client to problem solve by working through solutions and stating the options. The therapist frequently confronts the client with the consequences of his or her behavior and assigns homework problems for the client to try out new behaviors.

Reality Orientation. Treatment that assists confused patients in understanding the current situation. For example, during a treatment group, the therapist may have each patient give his or her name, the date, or the situation that brought the patient to the hospital. Discussion between the members of the group may help orient the patient to reality in a less threatening manner than if the therapist completes orientation. If the patient is being treated individually, the therapist may have a memory board posted that the patient uses each day to recite time and place. The therapist may then discuss the patient's situation and other personal items of concern. See Cognitive-perceptual deficits for further discussion and treatment.

Reality Therapy.   A Psychotherapy technique introduced by Glasser (1965) that focuses on helping the client take responsibility for his or her behavior and confront problems directly.

Rebound Phenomenon of Holmes.   Inability to control movements so that a contraction can be stopped quickly in order to avoid hitting an object. A patient who demonstrates this deficit will hit himself in the face or arm if the patient is flexing the elbow against the therapist's resistance and the resistance is quickly withdrawn without warning the patient.

Recognition.   The cognitive ability to identify familiar faces and objects. It is based on the individual's ability to retrieve memory. Activities to aid memory include cue cards.

Reductionism.   Reducing complex situations, data, phenomena, and experiences to simple terms. An example is to treat major depression, a complex illness that affects an individual's ability to Work, socialize with others, engage in Leisure activities, and regulate one's Self-care by taking a drug to relieve symptoms. A holistic approach is in contrast to reductionistic treatment.

Reflex.   An involuntary muscle response to sensory stimuli. Some reflexes occur during infancy and disappear later, for example, the Asymmetrical tonic neck, Moro reflex, Neck-righting, Rooting, Stepping, and Sucking. Other reflexes are purposeful in the adult such as flexor withdrawal, postural proprioception, and pupillary.

Reflexes and Reactions.   As an infant, sensory stimulation can evoke automatic movements. As motor development occurs, these automatic movements become integrated by the central nervous system. CNS integration allows a person to move voluntarily rather than being governed by those automatic movements. However, if a person sustains a brain injury, the person may revert to automatic movements based on the location of brain insult. McCormack and Feuchter (1996) and Mathiowitz and Haugen (1995) listed the following locations of integration for some of the reflexes and reactions:

Locations of Integration

- **Spinal Level**: Extensor thrust, flexor withdrawal, crossed extension, negative supporting reaction, Grasp, and cutaneous fusimotor reflexes (McCormack & Feuchter, 1996, also placed Positive supporting reaction in this category).

- **Brain Stem Level**: Tonic labyrinthine reflex (TLR), tonic neck reflexes (TNRs), tonic lumbar reflexes, and associated reactions (Mathiowitz & Haugen, 1995, also placed Positive supporting reaction in this category).

- **Midbrain/Cortical Level**: Body on body righting, body and head righting, labyrinthine righting, neck righting, optical righting, protective extension, and equilibrium reactions.

- **Cortical Level**: Higher level voluntary movement

Below is a list of reflexes and reactions that can be observed as developmental milestones in children, but some of them may also be demonstrated by a person who has had a stroke or other insult to the brain. The general time for integration is listed to help the therapist determine if a child is delayed in development. A diagnosis of delay should not be based solely on the integration of reflexes and reactions. The therapist should utilize pediatric tests of development such as the *Bayley Scales of Infant Development—II* (Bayley, 1993), *Peabody Developmental Motor Scales* (Folio & Fewell, 1983), or the *Bruininks-Oseretsky Test of Motor Proficiency* (Bruininks, 1978) to measure a child's performance in different areas.

Developmental Reflexes

- **Oral Reflexes**
  - *Rooting*: When a child's skin is stroked at the corner of the mouth, the child turns his or her head toward the side being stimulated. This reflex begins at birth, and integration occurs between 2–3 months of age.

- *Suck-swallow*: When liquid is presented to a child, the child sucks and reflexively swallows. This reflex begins at birth, and integration occurs around 4 months of age.
- *Bite*: When a child's gums are touched with an object, the child bites down on the object. This reflex begins near 4 months of age and integration occurs around 7 months of age.
- *Gag*: When pressure is applied on the middle-to-back of the child's tongue, the child grimaces, constricts the pharynx, and thrusts the tongue. This reflex begins at birth, and it exists throughout the lifespan. As a child, the reflex occurs more forward on the tongue and moves back as a person gets older.
- *Palatal*: When the faucial arches are stroked, the arches constrict and the uvula elevates. This reflex begins at birth and exists throughout the lifespan. It helps protect a person's airway and produce swallowing.

- **Moro Reflex**: A child is held in supine and the child's head is allowed to suddenly drop backward 20–30°. The head is then supported again. The response to the stimulus will first be abduction and extension of the child's arms, followed by flexion, adduction, and crossing of the arms across the body. This reflex begins at birth, and integration occurs around 5–6 months of age.
- **Palmar Grasp Reflex**: When an adult places a finger (or object) into a child's palm from the ulnar side, the fingers flex and grasp the adult's finger. This reflex begins at birth, and integration occurs around 2 months of age.
- **Plantar Grasp Reflex**: When an adult places pressure on the sole of a child's foot, the toes flex around the adult's hand (or object being used). This reflex begins at birth, and integration occurs around 12 months of age.
- **Positive Supporting Reaction**: When a child is positioned with the ball of the foot in contact with a surface, the leg will extend and bear some weight. This reflex begins at birth, and integration occurs around 6 months of age. If a patient exhibits this reflex following a brain

injury, he or she will have difficulty with ambulation and transfers since the affected leg will want to rigidly extend whenever it contacts a surface.

- **Automatic Stepping**. When a child is held in a slightly forward position so that the soles of both feet are in firm contact with a surface, the legs will make rhythmical and alternating stepping movements. This reflex begins at birth, and integration occurs around 2 months of age.

- **Placing Response or Placing Reaction**: When a child's palm comes into contact with a hard surface, the patient will bear weight on that extremity. This reflex begins at birth, and integration occurs around 2 months of age.

- **Tonic Neck Reflexes (TNR)**: A brainstem level reflex present early in life but may return due to a brain injury. A child or patient demonstrates this reflex when the position of the person's neck affects the person's limbs. This reflex has been further subdivided into an assymetrical tonic neck reflex (ATNR) and a symmetrical tonic neck reflex (STNR)

  - *Asymmetrical Tonic Neck Reflex (ATNR)*: When a child's head is turned 90° to one side, he or she extends the upper extremity nearest the face, and flexes the upper extremity nearest the back of the head. This reflex is present at birth, and integration occurs around 4–6 months of age. A patient who has had a brain injury may also exhibit this reflex. When a patient's head is turned 90° to one side, he or she demonstrates an increase in extensor tone of the upper extremity nearest the face, and an increase in flexor tone of the upper extremity nearest the back of the head. If a patient exhibits this reflex, he or she will have difficulty moving the affected arm voluntarily since movement will be dependent on the his or her head position.

  - *Symmetrical Tonic Neck Reflex (STNR)*: When a child's head is flexed, the child demonstrates flexion of the arms and extension of the legs. Likewise, when the child's head is extended, the child demonstrates extension of the arms and flexion of the legs. This reflex is present at birth, and integration occurs around 4–6 months of age. If a patient who has had a brain injury exhibits this reflex, he or she will have difficulty transferring from sitting to standing since his or her legs will extend when the head flexes.

- **Tonic Lumbar Reflex**: When a child's chest is rotated to the right, the child flexes the right upper extremity and extends the right lower extremity. Simultaneously, the left upper extremity extends and the left lower extremity flexes. This reflex is present at birth, and integration occurs at 4–6 months of age. A patient who had had a brain injury may have difficulty voluntarily controlling the affected extremities if this reflex is present.

- **Landau Reflex**: When a child is supported at the stomach while in prone, the hips, back, and neck extend. This reflex begins to form at birth but is not complete until 6 months of age. Integration occurs at 10–12 months of age.

- **Galant Reflex**: When the child is stroked along one side of the vertebrae, the spine will flex or curve toward the side being stimulated. This reflex begins at birth.

- **Crossed Extension**: When a child is in supine, one leg begins in extension while the other is in flexion. As the extended leg is flexed, the flexed leg will extend, adduct, and internally rotate. This reflex begins at birth, and integration occurs around 2 months of age. If a patient exhibits this reflex, he or she will have difficulty with ambulation since abnormal extension will occur in the affected leg when the unaffected leg is flexing.

- **Flexor Withdrawal**: When the sole of a child's foot is tickled or pricked, the leg receiving the stimulus will flex to withdraw from the stimulus. This reflex begins at birth, and integration occurs around 2 months of age.

- **Extensor Thrust**: The child begins with one leg flexed. When the sole of the foot of the flexed leg is stroked, the leg extends. This reflex begins at birth, and integration occurs around 2 months of age.

- **Tonic Labyrinthine Reflexes (TLR)**: This brainstem level reflex is present early in life but may return due to a brain injury. A patient demonstrates this reflex when the position of the patient's trunk influences movement. This reflex can be subdivided into a *tonic labyrinthine supine reflex (TLS)* and a *tonic labyrinthine prone reflex (TLP)*. If a patient exhibits this reflex, he or she will have difficulty going from supine to sitting. Extensor tone will make trunk flexion difficult at first. Then as forward movement occurs, flexor tone will increase and put the patient at risk for falling forward off the bed.

  - *Tonic Labyrinthine Supine Reflex (TLS)*: When a child is placed in supine (the neck is usually flexed), both upper and lower extremities extend. This reflex begins at birth, and integration occurs around 4 months of age.
  - *Tonic Labyrinthine Prone Reflex (TLP)*: When a child is placed is prone (the neck is usually extended), both upper and lower extremities flex. This reflex begins at birth, and integration occurs around 4 months of age.

- **Grasp Reflex**: The application of deep pressure (of the therapist's hand) to the child's palm results in digit flexion and adduction, or a closing of the fist. This is also referred to as Palmar grasp reflex (see above). The patient will not be able to open his or her hand, even if able to actively extend the fingers of the affected hand. This reflex is used to elicit movement when treating with the Brunnstrom approach. See Motor control problems, Movement therapy of Brunnstrom.

- **Babkins Reflex**: When pressure is applied to a child's palms, the child's mouth opens. This reflex begins at birth, and integration occurs around 4 months of age.

- **Babinski Reflex**: A stimulus (such as a light stroke) is presented to the plantar surface of the foot which results in dorsiflexion of the great toe. This reflex occurs when the upper motor neuron tracts of the spinal cord are interrupted before reaching the lumbosacral reflex center. This reflex may be demonstrated by a patient who has had a stroke, spinal cord injury, or multiple sclerosis.

- **Finger Extension**: When the child's ulnar border of the hand is stroked, the fingers extend and the hand opens.
- **Deep Tendon Reflexes**: Reaction of the tendons of specific muscles to a tap resulting in a slight and quick jerk. For example, the test for the quadriceps is completed by the physician tapping on the tendon distal to the patella resulting in a knee jerk. Other commonly tested tendons include the biceps brachii, brachioradialis, triceps brachii, and gastrocnemius-soleus. Deep tendon reflexes are tested to help check for symptoms of Upper motor neuron disorders.
- **Associated Reactions**: When voluntary movement in a child's limb is resisted, the opposite limb moves involuntarily. For example, if the therapist resists shoulder flexion with the left upper extremity, the right upper extremity will flex at the shoulder. This reflex begins at birth, and integration occurs between 8–9 years of age.

Reactions

- **Optical Righting**: When a child is tilted so that the body is no longer vertical, the head will right itself so that it remains vertical. This reaction begins around 2 months of age, and it continues throughout the lifespan.
- **Labyrinthine Righting**: When a child is tilted so that the body is no longer vertical, the head will right itself to the vertical position, even though the patient's eyes are covered so that visual cues cannot be used to orient the head. This reaction begins around 2 months of age, and it continues throughout the lifespan.
- **Neck Righting**: When a child's head is turned to one side, the body rolls to that same side at the same time. The head and body cannot roll separately from one another, so the patient "log-rolls." This reaction begins at

birth, and integration occurs around 6 months of age.

- **Body Righting on Body**: When a child's head is turned to one side, the body is able to roll segmentally. The upper trunk rolls first, and the pelvis and lower extremities follow. This reflex may also be referred to as body on body righting. This reaction begins at 6 months, and integration occurs around 18 months.

- **Body Righting on Head**: When a part of the body is touching a supporting surface, the head adjusts to a vertical position. For example, when a child is lying prone, the neck flexes so that the head is lifted to between 45–90° vertical. Likewise, when a child is lying supine, the neck extends to lift the head. This reaction begins at 1–2 months of age when the child is prone, and 5–6 months of age when the child is supine.

- **Protective Arm Extension**: A reaction of the extremities during an Equilibrium reaction. If equilibrium cannot be reestablished by the body, then the extremities will automatically abduct and/or extend to protect the body when falling. Protective arm extension occurs in a forward direction, lateral direction, and backward direction. This reaction begins at 6 months of age for both forward and lateral extension, but it is not present in the backward direction until 9 months of age. It continues throughout the lifespan.

- **Equilibrium Reactions**: A reaction of the body to shift its center of gravity to maintain balance when a supporting surface is moved. During the equilibrium reaction, Righting of the head and upper trunk can be observed as well as Protective reactions of extremities. A child learns to use equilibrium reactions while in prone, supine, quadruped, sitting, and standing. These reactions begin between 6–21 months, and they continue throughout the lifespan.

Reflexology.   The application of massage of reflex points on feet and hands to encourage health and well being.

Reflexes and Reactions

Reflex Sympathetic Dystrophy Syndrome (RSD).
A disorder that results in pain, edema, and sympathetic nervous system dysfunction that is much worse than expected from the patient's original condition (such as nerve injury). The exact cause is unknown; however, the syndrome often occurs following trauma, nerve injury, or a central nervous system disorder. This disorder may be classified into the following types of RSD:
- Shoulder-hand syndrome
- Causalgia
- Neurovascular dystrophy
- Sudeck's atrophy
- Idiopathic peripheral autonomic neuropathy
- Posttraumatic dystrophy
- Algodystrophy.

Onset most often occurs between the ages of 45–65 years of age, and this disorder is more common in women.

    Treatment. One specific treatment technique for this disorder is *stress loading*. Compression activities, such as scrubbing a floor while on the hands and knees, should be completed for 3 minutes, three times a day. The patient should also complete traction activities, such as carrying a weighted briefcase in the affected hand, throughout the day.

Regression. Relapse or exacerbation of symptoms in which an individual's illness gets worse. For example, an individual who is making improvement from an episode of depression suddenly regresses with exaggerated feelings of suicide.

Rehabilitation. The restoration of function in an individual with an acquired disability. Function relates to competence in an individual's ability to work, to be independent in <u>Self-care</u> and <u>Leisure</u> activities, and to have the social skills for effective personal interactions.

Reinforcement Schedule. The method of reinforcing a client's behavior. This can be on a ratio or interval schedule to help a client to learn or maintain a task or behavior. For example, in a ratio schedule, a client is reinforced for completion of a specific task (e.g., tying a shoelace or demonstrating positive interactions). In an interval schedule, the client is reinforced for appropriate behavior based on a time interval, such as every 15 minutes or half-hour.

Relaxation Response.   A treatment method developed by Herbert Benson (1975) based originally on transcendental meditation. In this method the client is taught to have a passive attitude and to recite a verbal phrase to him- or herself while in a comfortable position. The physiological reaction that is sought is produced by sitting serenely and alone in a quiet place with eyes closed and arms and hands relaxed; paying careful attention to breathing; and repeating a brief word or phrase at each respiratory cycle. The aim is to reach a tranquil mental state that refreshes the mind and body. It is recommended that the client practice the technique every day and to incorporate it into his or her schedule.

Relaxation Therapy.   Techniques that help an individual to reduce bodily tension, anxiety, heart rate, blood pressure and overall sympathetic responses that occur when an individual is overaroused. In designing a relaxation program the therapist should consider the following:

- The purposes of the program, such as reducing the individual's anxiety so that he or she will be better able to work, engage in leisure activities, or be independent in Self-care.
- The context of the therapy such as group or individual sessions, number and length of sessions, and environment where sessions will take place.
- The specific therapies used such as Relaxation response, Progressive relaxation, Visualization, or meditation.
- The evaluation of the relaxation experience through client evaluation, standardized test or physiological measure.

Remission.   The lessening of symptoms or complete recovery from an illness. For example in an individual diagnosed

Remission. *(continued)*

with Schizophrenia, the symptoms of hallucinations and Delusions may disappear and the individual is able to work and engage in normal activities. Individuals may be in remission for weeks, months, or years.

Resting tremor. See Tremor.

Retrograde Massage. A technique used to help reduce and control edema. See Edema for further discussion and treatment method.

Rett's Syndrome. A genetic condition that progresses from impaired hand function to ataxia, autistic characteristics, language problems, and dementia.

Reversal of Antagonists. A technique which was used by Voss (1967) during treatment within the framework of PNF. The supporting theory states that a stronger antagonist can help facilitate a weaker agonist (Sherrington, 1961). Resistance is given to the antagonist to help promote contraction of the agonist. Three specific techniques include slow reversal, slow reversal-hold, and rhythmic stabilization. See Motor control problems, Proprioceptive neuromuscular facilitation for more discussion of these techniques.

Reye Syndrome. A condition which occurs after a patient has contracted a virus. Symptoms begin with vomiting and can proceed to cognitive impairments such as disorientation, lethargy, and possibly a coma. Death can also occur from edema of the brain that may cause cerebral herniation.

Rheumatoid Arthritis. A systemic disease that results in inflammation of the joints (especially the synovial lining), that can destroy surrounding joint structures. Rheumatoid arthritis occurs in remissions and exacerbations. Symptoms include pain, morning stiffness, fatigue, muscle wasting, anemia, and decreased movement of the affected joints.

The cause is unknown, and onset usually occurs between the ages of 25–50 years of age.

Specific Treatments

- Complete activities to maintain ROM, strength, and endurance
- Fabricate splints to prevent deformity: a resting hand Splint or a splint to prevent ulnar deviation are indicated for a person with this diagnosis
- Recommend the use of knee extension splints at night
- Instruct the patient on pain management techniques
- Educate the patient on the importance of avoiding fatigue or overexertion
- Teach the patient to use energy conservation, work simplification, and especially joint protection principles during activities
- Encourage the patient to join a support group to assist with emotional adjustment to the disease
- Provide education on assistive devices to increase the patient's independence with Self-care activities as needed
- Complete a home evaluation and give recommendations to improve the patient's mobility in the home as well as ability to continue functional tasks such as laundry or cooking
- Help the patient modify Leisure activities as needed or explore new leisure interests

Contraindications/Precautions

- Stress the importance of compliance with joint protection, energy conservation, and work simplification principles to prevent deformity
- Monitor for skin breakdown from Splints
- Avoid overexertion
- Monitor for symptoms of Carpal tunnel syndrome

Right-Left Discrimination. The perceptual process or ability to differentiate between the right and left sides of

Right-Left Discrimination. *(continued)*
the body. Individuals with Learning disabilities can have
difficulty with this skill. See Cognitive-perceptual deficits
for further discussion and treatment.

Righting Reaction. A reaction of the body to gain normal
alignment between the head and trunk or extremities, or to
position the head in its normal upright position in space (so
that the head is vertical and the mouth is horizontal). For
specific reactions, see Reflexes and reactions.

Rigidity. Hypertonicity of both agonist and antagonist
muscles so that resistance to passive movement can be felt
in any direction or at any point in the range of motion.
Types of Rigidity
- **Cogwheel Rigidity**: Characterized by a rhythmic relaxation and contraction of muscles during passive movement. When moving a body part with cogwheel rigidity,
the part may be difficult to move at first, but then both
agonist and antagonist muscles will relax so that movement is easier. However, the muscle Cocontraction will
again occur, making movement difficult. This contracting
and relaxing will occur many times while the therapist
moves the part through its ROM, so that movement feels
like it keeps "catching."
- **Lead Pipe Rigidity**: Characterized by *constant* resistance
to movement in any direction with no relaxation of the
agonist or antagonist muscles occurring. This hypertonicity is uniform so that the same resistance is felt at
any point in the affected joint's ROM.

Rocking. A technique used to either facilitate or inhibit
Muscle tone. If completed in a fast manner, rocking produces vestibular stimulation, which helps facilitate tone. If
completed in a slow manner, rocking helps inhibit tone so
that a spastic muscle relaxes through a wider range of
motion. See Motor control problems, Rood approach for
further discussion of facilitation and inhibition techniques.

Role Performance. A social component that includes the individual's position in a family, job, culture, nation, or religion. These role functions include husband/wife, occupational title, political leader, spiritual counselor, parent/homemaker, and professional soldier. These role functions are gained through education and social and family expectations. Throughout one's life, role functions are assumed and changed. Occupational therapists can help clients to gain insight into their various role performances and develop new roles (e.g., volunteering, changing jobs, becoming a better parent). Use of role performance tests, counseling, and Role playing are used to assist the client.

Role Playing. Simulation of family, work, social, interpersonal, or community situations. The client portrays roles in previous situations (e.g., conflicts) and in future situations (e.g., applying for a job). The therapist provides a supportive environment and coaching to help the client increase social skills. Can also be used in a Group therapy context where other clients can give feedback and consensual validation. The therapist can also use role reversal to help clients gain insight into roles.

Rolfing. The application of deep massage to the connective tissue, which is the wrapping that binds and connects muscles and bones (Rolf, 1977). The purpose of rolfing is to increase the range of motion of the joints and to enhance suppleness by stretching and unwinding the fascia, which become thickened and stuck together causing pain and immobility in the client. The massage involves deep sliding movements to the neck, shoulder, torso, and lower extremities.

Rolling. A technique that can help decrease high muscle tone. The patient assumes a sidelying position on the uninvolved side. The therapist sits behind the patient and places his or her hands on the patient's affected hip and shoulder/rib cage. The therapist slowly rolls the patient from side

Rolling. *(continued)*
lying into prone and back to side lying, with a slow rhythmic motion. A pillow under the patient's head or between the knees may be necessary to preserve alignment during this activity. Rolling should be completed first with the patient side lying on the nonaffected side, and then side lying on the affected side. See Motor control problems, Rood approach for further discussion of inhibition techniques.

Romberg's Sign. A test that examines the proprioceptive function of the dorsal columns.
- The patient is asked to stand with heels together while keeping the eyes open.
- The therapist should observe how much the patient sways, and then ask the patient to maintain balance while closing the eyes and keeping the feet together.
- If the patient sways much more or even nearly falls when the eyes are shut, this is a positive Romberg's sign that the dorsal columns, which are responsible for proprioception, are affected by injury or disease.
- A patient who has cerebellar dysfunction will sway equally or more when the eyes are open.

Rood Approach. A traditional approach to the treatment of a person who has difficulty controlling movement. This treatment is based on the premise that sensory stimuli can normalize abnormal muscle tone, which helps elicit motor responses. Sensory stimuli can be used for the facilitation or inhibition of muscle tone. Other important principles include the following: motor control returns in a developmental sequence, and treatment should focus on the *goal* of a movement rather than the movement itself, since the nervous system is able to automatically elicit the correct movement to reach a specific goal. See Motor control problems, Rood approach for more specific methods of treatment.

Rotator Cuff Muscles. The four muscles that attach around the shoulder joint and help form a musculotendinous cuff to help hold the head of the humerus in the glenoid fossa. These muscles include the supraspinatus, infraspinatus, teres minor, and subscapularis. See Appendix D for a table of the muscles of the body including their origins, insertions, actions, and innervations.

Rowing. A technique used to facilitate elbow extension within Brunnstrom's (1970, 1996) framework of movement therapy to regain motor control.
- The therapist sits facing the patient with his or her arms pronated, extended at the elbows, and crossed at the wrists.
- The patient has his or her arms supinated and flexed at the elbows.
- The therapist places his or her hands in the patient's palms.
- The therapist asks the patient to help actively extend the elbows while the therapist assists.
- As the therapist flexes his or her elbows and supinates his or her forearms (which results in the therapist uncrossing his or her arms), the patient extends his or her elbows while pronating and crossing his or her arms at the wrists.
- The therapist should use resist the noninvolved arm as it moves into elbow extension to help produce an associated reaction in the involved arm. See Reflexes and reactions.
- The therapist should have the patient relax as the therapist passively guides the patient's arms back into flexion and supination, while the therapist returns to elbows extended, forearms pronated and crossed at the wrists.

See Motor control problems, Movement therapy of Brunnstrom.

RUMBA. An acronym for Relevant, Understandable, Measurable, Behavioral and Achievable. It is used as a guide in writing operational treatment objectives for clients.

Sagittal plane. See Anatomical position.

Scapula Abduction. Movement of the scapula away from the spine. The preferred term for Scapula protraction; however, Bobath (1978) referred to protraction when discussing treatment techniques.

Scapula Adduction. Movement of the scapula toward the spine. Currently, this term is preferred over scapula retraction.

Scapula Depression. A gliding movement of the scapula downward or away from the patient's head.

Scapula Elevation. A gliding movement of the scapula upward or toward the patient's head.

Scapula Protraction. The act of bringing the scapula forward around the ribcage, which naturally occurs when a person reaches forward. Bobath (1978) stressed the importance of the therapist passively completing this motion when a patient demonstrates a flexor synergy. Treatment must begin proximally and move distally. Scapula abduction is currently the preferred term for this motion. See Motor control problems, Neurodevelopmental treatment for more treatment techniques.

Scapula Retraction. See Scapula adduction.

Scapular Mobilization. A technique, specifically referred to by Bobath (1978), used to help maintain the glide of the scapulothoracic joint and allow the extremity its full range of motion. This is often completed while the patient is in supine, but it can also be completed with the patient in a sidelying or sitting position. The therapist places one hand on the patient's scapula and the other hand on the patient's proximal humerus to help externally rotate the humerus during this activity. The therapist then elevates/depresses and abducts/adducts the scapula with the patient's arm at 0° flexion. If the scapula glides freely, the arm may be flexed to

30°–60° while completing the same gliding motions. If there is still no resistance to gliding, the arm is flexed to near 90° during the same gliding motions. When the scapula demonstrates glide in all three positions, the therapist may proceed to passive shoulder range of motion through full range. See Motor control problems, Neurodevelopmental treatment for more treatment techniques.

Scapulohumeral Rhythm. The coordination of the scapulothoracic, glenohumeral, acromioclavicular, and sternoclavicular joints to produce 60° of scapulothoracic movement and 120° of glenohumeral movement which allows a full 180° of range of motion at the shoulder. If one of these joints is disrupted, then the combined scapula-humerus motion will be inhibited and shoulder movement will be decreased. Scapula mobilization should be completed prior to range of motion activities, especially if the patient has abnormal muscle tone, to make sure that the scapula is gliding along the rib cage and not inhibiting shoulder motion.

Schizoid Personality Disorder. Symptomatic of individuals who are withdrawn, introspective, oversensitive, seclusive, and detached from initiating and maintaining close relationships. The individual with a schizoid personality disorder tends to working alone and has difficulty in expressing feelings. Treatment includes Social skills training, Role playing, and Creative expression.

Schizophrenia. A severe psychotic mental disorder affecting approximately 1% of the population that can be classified into subtypes such as paranoid, catatonic, disorganized, undifferentiated, and residual. A diagnosis of schizophrenia is made if symptoms such as delusions, hallucinations, thinking disorders, and disorganized behavior are present for at least 6 months. The symptoms of schizophrenia interfere with the individual's ability to carry out the normal role functions in Work, Leisure, Self-care, and social interactions.

There are several theories to explain the cause or causes of schizophrenia.

- Genetic factors which assumes that the individual has inherited a vulnerability or tendency towards introversion, social withdrawal, and a low threshold for coping with stress.
- Biochemical theories which assume that individuals with schizophrenia have neurological impairments such as high levels of dopamine in the brain, which leads to hyper-arousal, or structural differences in the ventricles of the brain.
- Psychological theories based on developmental factors in the individual such as family relationships where high expressed emotion may cause the individual to have low-ered self-esteem and ability to cope with everyday problems of living.
- Sociocultural theories relate to the factors such as impoverishment, poverty, class prejudice, and social disorganization that leads to severe anxiety, inadequacy, passive dependence and alienation.
- Eclectic theories assume that there is a multifactorial nature to schizophrenia where genetic, biochemical, psychological and sociocultural factors interact to cause a schizophrenic illness.

Symptoms of schizophrenia are characterized as either positive or negative. Positive symptoms include the addition or exaggerating of normal functions such as visual or auditory hallucinations, delusional thinking, or disorganized speech or behavior. Negative symptoms on the other hand reflect a loss of function such as social withdrawal, lack of affect, apathy, and low motivation

Types of Schizophrenia

- **Disorganized**, that is, characterized by a complete breakdown in social relationships, incoherence, and bizarre personalized behavior.
- **Catatonic,** in which an individual displays psychomotor disturbances ranging from rigidity to frenetic activity

- **Paranoid ideation,** dominating individual's interaction with others
- **Undifferentiated,** where no one symptom dominates behavior
- **Residual** is the mildest type of schizophrenia where the major symptoms include social isolation, inappropriate affects, and eccentric behavior.

Course of Illness. The first symptoms of schizophrenia usually occur during early adolescence. About one third of individuals with one episode of symptoms of schizophrenia recover completely, another third of individuals require continuous treatment and respond well to medication and Cognitive-behavioral therapy while another third seems to be resistant to treatment and remain in an institution for the remainder of their lives.

Treatment

- Holistic approach is usually the most effective (Stein & Cutler, 1998)
- Medication such as clozopine, which is an antipsychotic drug, reduces the positive symptoms.
- Social skills training in attention and listening skills, ability to converse, being supportive, problem solving, and self-assessment.
- Stress management training in developing coping skills to manage the symptoms of stress and the situations that trigger stressful reactions.
- Leisure skills training, identifying leisure activities that the individual enjoys and can gain gratification through incorporating into everyday schedule.
- Exercise prescription to increase general well-being of individual and to control depression.
- Nutritional counseling to help individual identify foods that are enjoyable and healthy to increases quality of life.
- Housing referral to help individual to locate housing arrangement such as halfway house, a transitional

apartment, or foster care that enables an individual to be maximally independent.

- Support groups to give the individual an opportunity to express feelings and thought without critical judgments while developing reality testing.
- Creative arts to give the individual opportunities to develop specialized skills and interests in music, art, poetry, literature, ceramics, weaving, computers, and jewelry making.
- Counseling and Psychotherapy including individual or group therapy in which where the mental health professional works in alliance with individual in solving problems of everyday living including family conflicts.
- Vocational programming to help an individual gain vocational skills, experience in working, and placement in appropriate jobs.
- Family therapy and conflict resolution into individual's illness to help family members to gain insight.

Specific Occupational Therapy Guideline

- Develop a therapeutic alliance with individual based on mutual trust
- Help individual to incorporate activities, such as exercise, health, nutrition, medication, Creative arts, Leisure, and social skills into daily schedule.
- Encourage individual to monitor behavior and to ask for help when relapses may occur.
- Develop an individualized Stress management program
- Focus on strengths of individual

Seasonal Affective Disorder (SAD). A mood disorder accompanied by symptoms of depression such as fatigue, diminished concentration, sadness, sleep and eating disturbances, and a general malaise. It is thought to be caused by the diminishing of daytime sun in late fall and winter. Treatment includes light therapy, medication, Stress management, and exercise.

Secondary Prevention.   Prevention of the recurrence of a disease, for example, preventing a second stroke in an individual.

Self.   The individual's typical characteristics or personality that constitutes his or her identity. It is comprised of the affective, cognitive, and spiritual qualities that are distinctive.

Self-care.   Activities that are completed daily to maintain good hygiene and good appearance, meet basic needs such as eating and voiding, and move from one necessary area (such as the kitchen) to another (the bathroom). These basic required activities can be grouped together in a category also referred to as Activities of daily living (ADLs). Below are the subcategories of activities included in this area. Each subcategory contains adaptive techniques helpful to patients who exhibit impairments with specific performance components. Also refer to specific diagnoses/conditions within this guide for more treatment ideas. See Assistive technology for a list of devices that may assist patients with Self-care activities.

Dressing.   A Self-care activity that includes the following: retrieving clothing, appropriate for weather and time of year from storage areas; donning/doffing items in the proper sequence (socks before shoes); fastening all pieces of clothing, including shoes; and donning/doffing prostheses or orthoses.

- **Donning a Shirt**
  - *Method I (button-down shirt)*: The patient should grab the shirt by the collar and lay it across the lap so that it is inside out with the collar up by the stomach. The patient first opens the armhole nearest the affected arm and places the affected arm in it. Then the unaffected arm is placed in its armhole. Care should be taken to push the sleeve above the elbow on the affected arm. The patient then gathers the shirt and grasps it

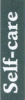

by the collar. While ducking the head, the patient uses the unaffected arm to pull the shirt over the head. The shirt is then pulled down in back and the buttons are fastened. To remove the shirt, the same steps are completed in reverse order. The shirt is first gathered up at the collar and pulled forward over the head. The final step is to remove the affected arm from the shirt.

- ***Method II (button-down shirt)***: The shirt is positioned on the lap as in Method I. The patient places the affected arm into the shirt first. The patient then grasps the shirt by the collar and pulls it around behind the back. The unaffected arm is then placed into the shirt, and the buttons are fastened. Again, to remove the shirt, the steps are completed in reverse so that the unaffected arm is removed first. The final step is to remove the affected arm.

- ***Method III (button-down shirt)***: The patient can first button the shirt while it is laying on his or her lap, and then use the method for donning a pullover shirt. The shirt is also removed by reversing the pullover shirt method.

- ***Method IV (pullover shirt)***: The patient positions the shirt so that the bottom hem is nearest the patient's stomach and the back side of the shirt is up. The patient then places the affected arm in the shirt and uses the unaffected arm to pull the sleeve on up past the elbow. Next, the patient places the unaffected arm in its armhole. The patient then gathers the back of the shirt and grasps it at the collar while pulling it over the head. The final step is to adjust the shirt in the back. To remove a pullover shirt, the method is reversed so that the shirt is first gathered up to the collar and pulled forward over the head.

- **Donning a Brassiere**
  - ***Method I (back-fastener)***: The patient can tuck one end of the brassiere into the pants' waistband while

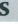
pulling the other end around the waist. The patient should then hook the brassiere and pull the fastener around to the back. The affected arm is placed through the arm strap, and the strap is pulled up onto the shoulder. The unaffected arm is then placed through the strap and positioned correctly. The brassiere is removed in the reverse order.

- *Method II (back fastener)*: The patient can fasten the brassiere while it is laying on her lap, and then don it over the head. After it has been fastened, the affected arm is placed through its strap. The unaffected arm is also placed through its strap, and then the back piece of the garment near the fastener is grasped and pulled overhead. The patient must than pull the brassier down completely in front and back. The brassiere should be removed in the reverse order. If the brassiere is too tight to easily be pulled down, a bra extension can be sewn onto the garment to increase its elasticity around the patient's middle.

- *Method III (sports bra)*: A bra can be purchased which is very elastic and has no fastener. This bra should be donned overhead, as was done in Method II.

- *Method IV (front fastener)*: The patient should first place the affected arm through its strap and pull it completely onto the shoulder. Next, the patient places the unaffected arm through its strap and pulls it onto the shoulder. The front of the bra should be positioned with the affected arm stabilizing that end of the garment. The patient then uses the unaffected arm to fasten the brassiere. The garment is removed in the reverse order.

- **Donning Pants**
  - *Method I*: The patient positions the pants on the lap with the affected leghole in front of the affected leg and the unaffected leghole in front of the unaffected leg. The patient then crosses the affected leg over the

unaffected leg at the knee, with help of the unaffected arm if needed. If unable to cross at the knee, the patient may cross the legs at the ankle. The patient places the affected leg through the leghole and pulls the pants completely over the foot while pulling the waistband only up to the knee. This allows the patient to place the unaffected leg into its leghole. The patient then pulls the pants completely over the unaffected foot and pulls the waistband as close to the hips as possible. If the pants do not have an elastic waist, the patient may place the pocket or beltloop in the affected hand to prevent the pants from falling to the floor while the patient stands. The patient then stands and pulls the pants to the waist. If the pants are large enough and the patient demonstrates good balance, the patient should fasten the button while standing. The patient can then fasten the zipper after sitting again. When removing the pants, complete the previous steps in the reverse order.

- *Method II*: The patient uses the previous method to place the legs into the legholes. Instead of standing, the patient extends the hips by pushing against the back of the chair and using the unaffected leg to push against the floor. While the hips are elevated from the seat, the patient pulls the pants to the waist and fastens the button if possible. The patient then fastens the zipper when sitting against the seat. The pants are removed in the reverse order.

- *Method III*: The patient completes this method while in bed. If possible, the head should be slightly elevated to assist the patient in reaching the feet. The patient first places the affected leg in the pants by crossing the leg over the unaffected leg or by bending the affected leg. The patient then places the unaffected leg in the pants. The patient uses the unaffected leg and arm to push against the bed and lift the bottom from the bed while pulling the pants to the waist. The patient can then lie against the bed while fastening the pants. When removing the pants, complete these steps in reverse.

- **Donning Socks**
  - The patient should cross the affected leg over the unaffected leg at the knee if possible. If the patient is not able to do this, the legs can also be crossed at the ankles. The patient then opens the end of the sock and pulls it onto the foot. The patient can insert the unaffected hand and spread the fingers apart in order to get the toes into the sock. Once the toes are completely in the sock, the patient can pull the sock over the heel and up into place. The patient then dons the sock onto the unaffected foot in the same manner. When removing the socks, complete the steps in the reverse order.

- **Donning Shoes**
  - The patient can slip the toes on the affected foot into the shoe if the patient can plantarflex enough to point the toes slightly. The patient should then cross the affected leg over the unaffected leg to pull the shoe onto the heel. If the shoe needs to be fastened, this should also be completed while the legs are crossed. The patient then dons the shoe onto the unaffected foot.
  - If the patient is unable to plantarflex, the patient can don the shoe onto the affected toes while sitting and crossing the affected leg over the unaffected knee. Otherwise, the patient can stand to help position the toes into the shoe.
  - A patient who demonstrates good balance may be able to bend over and use the finger to help push the heel into the shoe.

- **Donning an Ankle-Foot Orthosis (AFO)**
  - The leg of the pants should be lifted up past the area where the AFO will be applied. The patient should lift

the affected leg while plantarflexing or allowing gravity to point the toes. The toes are then placed into the AFO which is placed in the shoe. The toes are slowly pushed into the shoe. The patient may lift the back of the AFO upward to assist with pushing the heel into the AFO/shoe, or the patient can push on the knee to help push the heel down. The patient should then fasten the velcro straps and lower the pant leg. If the patient is unable to bend over to fasten the straps, the patient can carefully cross the affected leg with the AFO over the knee of the unaffected leg to fasten the AFO.

- A patient with severe swelling in the foot will have difficulty placing the foot into the AFO while it is already in the shoe. This patient can attempt to don the AFO first, and then use the unaffected hand to help lift the leg to place the toes in the shoe. The patient will require a long-handled shoehorn to help push the heel into the shoe.

• Use adaptive equipment to assist with activities according to the patient's needs. See Assistive technology and specific diagnoses/condition for treatment ideas.

Grooming

A Self-care activity that includes the following: retrieving items necessary for maintaining good hygiene; washing, combing, and styling the hair; removing unwanted hair (shaving); caring for the nails; brushing the teeth or completing other mouth care; cleaning the ears; applying deodorant; and caring for other skin.

• A patient who demonstrates decreased endurance or back pain should sit to complete activities when possible.

• Assistance from another person may be needed to help a patient wash and style the hair or apply cosmetics.

• Labels can be placed on items to help the patient identify objects.

• Use adaptive equipment to assist with activities according to the patient's needs. See Assistive technology and specific diagnoses/condition for treatment ideas.

Feeding/Eating

A <u>Self-care</u> activity that includes washing hands before the meal; opening containers or other items that will be necessary during the meal (i.e., milk carton); using appropriate utensils and dishes; transferring food from the dish to the mouth; chewing and swallowing the food; cleaning oneself following the meal as needed; and managing other means of nutrition if needed (tube-feeding).

- The therapist should first check that the patient is positioned properly while eating for safety in swallowing.
- A coated spoon should be used if the patient has a tendency to clench the teeth following oral stimulation.
- The therapist may also complete an oral stimulation program to assist the patient with moving food around the mouth or desensitizing the patient from textures that are uncomfortable.
- Use adaptive equipment to assist with activities according to the patient's needs. See <u>Assistive technology</u> and specific diagnoses/condition for treatment ideas.
- High technology equipment is available for patients who have more impairments in function. A patient with quadriplegia, <u>Cerebral palsy</u>, <u>Multiple sclerosis</u>, and other neurological disabilities can benefit from an electric self-feeder that is operated through the use of a head or chin switch.

Transfers/Mobility

A <u>Self-care</u> activity which includes the ability to move throughout the living area, relocate from one piece of furniture to another, or position oneself within a piece of furniture (such as the bed).

- **Bed Mobility**
  - A patient should use the bedside rail to help assist the patient with rolling.
  - A patient with <u>Hemiplegia</u> usually demonstrates difficulty with rolling onto the unaffected side. The patient may be able to hook the unaffected leg under the affected leg to help bring it across the body. The

patient should also use the unaffected hand to grasp the affected hand and bring it across the body. These motions should assist the patient with rolling toward the unaffected side as well as lowering the lower extremities when attempting to sit at the edge of the bed.

- A trapeze can be installed above the patient's bed to assist the patient with pulling self up in bed.

- **Wheelchair Mobility**
  - A patient with Hemiplegia can learn to propel the wheelchair with the unaffected arm and leg. Patients who are demonstrate incoordination can use both feet to propel the wheelchair.
  - A patient with quadriplegia, spastic Cerebral palsy, or degenerative disease will benefit from an electric wheelchair. Training and practice will be important to the patient's progress in maneuvering the wheelchair.
  - A patient will require assistance when going up onto curbs, unless the patient is able to safely complete a "wheelie" while correctly distributing his or her weight to prevent a fall.

- **Transfers**
  - It is very important that the wheelchair should be locked during all transfers.
  - The patient should wear a transfer or gait belt during *all* transfers. This allows the therapist to hold onto the patient securely without pulling on a weak extremity. Staff should be taught this principle also, since patients with hemiplegia are at risk of injury of the affected extremities.
  - If the patient is unable to assist with the transfer, a lift should be used. If a lift is not available, the therapist may need to ask for assistance to perform a *two-person carry* transfer. Once a patient is in a sitting position, one person stands near the patient's head while the other stands nears the patient's feet. While using good

body mechanics, the lifter nearest the patient's head places the arms around the patient's chest from behind the patient and grasps one wrist with the opposite hand. The lifter nearest the patient's feet places his or her arms behind the patient's knees and grasps one wrist with the opposite hand. The lifters then lift the patient and move him or her to the desired target surface. If transferring the patient to a wheelchair, the lifter who is supporting the patient's upper body should carefully walk behind the back of the wheelchair to lower the patient nearest the back of the wheelchair.

- If the patient is unable to bear weight on the lower extremities but demonstrates fair upper extremity strength, a *sliding board transfer* can be completed. The board bridges the gap between the transfer surfaces. The board should be snugly placed under the patient's bottom with the opposite end of the board resting on the surface of the target chair or location. When possible, the patient should transfer toward the unaffected side. This allows the patient to use the strong arm to help pull oneself along the board toward the target surface.

- A patient who has good upper extremity strength can depress the scapulae to lift his bottom from a chair and pivot to another surface. This method is called a *depression transfer*. The transfer surfaces should be placed as close in proximity as possible during this transfer. The patient should remove the armrest of the wheelchair, if the patient is in a wheelchair, and place one arm on the target surface with the other arm on the surface from which the patient is transferring. The patient then depresses the scapulae while lifting the bottom off the chair and swings the bottom toward the target surface.

- A patient who is able to bear weight on the lower extremities can learn to *pivot transfer*, which requires very little, if any, ambulation. The patient should begin by transferring toward the unaffected side. The transfer surfaces should be placed in close proximity at a 90° angle, which allows the patient to go from one surface to another with only 1/4 turn. The patient should scoot to the edge of the chair. With verbal cues, the patient should attempt to stand while the therapist helps the patient to stand and pivot. The patient should push up from the armrests or surface from which the patient is transferring. The patient will have difficulty standing if the center of gravity is not brought over the patient's feet. The therapist should instruct the patient to bring the nose over the knees to help with this component. After turning, the patient should reach back for the armrests of the chair to which the patient is transferring. The patient should not sit down until the knees are resting against the seat. Once the patient has demonstrated knowledge of the transfer method, the patient should also learn to pivot transfer toward the affected side.

- A patient will complete a transfer easier if the surface he or she is transferring to is lower or the same height as the surface being transferred from.
- The therapist should be careful to observe good body mechanics while assisting a patient with a transfer to prevent injury of the therapist's back.

Bathing

A Self-care activity that includes retrieving items that will be used during the activity; transferring to and from the tub or shower; and soaping, rinsing, and drying oneself.

- The patient should never bathe if he or she is home alone until the patient has demonstrated consistent independence with all activities included in bathing.
- After bathing, the tub should be completely drained before the patient transfers out of the tub.
- If the patient demonstrates poor balance or safety, the therapist should encourage the patient to sponge bathe after returning home.

- Sliding glass doors should be removed and replaced with a shower curtain. This provides the patient with a larger area for transferring him- or herself to/from the tub.
- If a patient has a bathtub only, a hand-held shower can be purchased and easily attached to the faucet. This removes the need of the patient to get all of the way down into the tub.
- A patient may prefer baths and want to get into the tub after returning home. The therapist should then have the patient practice this transfer a few times before returning home to make sure the patient is able to do this. The therapist should also recommend grab bars.
- Use adaptive equipment to assist with activities according to the patient's needs. See <u>Assistive technology</u> and specific diagnoses/condition for treatment ideas.

Toileting

A <u>Self-care</u> activity that includes: retrieving items that will be used during the activity; transferring to and from the toilet; managing the clothing when sitting or standing; cleaning him- or herself after voiding; and caring for other needs, such as menstruation or incontinence.

- Stool softeners can be used to make bowel movements easier for a patient with poor endurance. Softeners may also be necessary to counteract the constipating side effects of some medications.
- A patient with poor safety judgment should not be left alone while on the toilet. The therapist should remain with the patient or stand right outside the door during toileting.
- Use adaptive equipment to assist with activities according to the patient's needs. See <u>Assistive technology</u> and specific diagnoses/condition for treatment ideas.

Self-Concept or Self-Image. An individual's perceptions, feelings, and attitudes about his or her own identity, values, capabilities, and weaknesses. It is an individual's assessment of self in regard to environmental mastery,

Self-care

Self-Concept or Self-Image. *(continued)*
ability to cope with stress, confidence in social situations, and ability to perform a job. Self-concept is determined by feedback from others, self-evaluations, and competence in performing tasks. Activities that ensure success for clients reinforces a positive self-concept and increases Self-esteem.

Self-Control. Modifying one's behavior in response to environmental needs, demands, constraints, personal aspirations, and feedback from others. Occupational therapists enable clients to self-regulate behaviors such as coping with stress, Time management, Pain management, Behavior modification, and Social skills training.

Self-Efficacy. An individual's perception of being able to perform a functional task or occupation.

Self-Esteem. Individual's appraisal of his or her competencies and abilities to succeed or master tasks that he or she is confronted with on a daily basis. An individual's self-esteem can be assessed as low or high depending on his or her self-confidence in performing a task.

Self-Evaluation Method. Subjects assess their own progress. Self-evaluation is an important factor in assessing treatment effectiveness. Other factors used in assessing treatment effectiveness include objective tests, psychophysiological measures, and mechanical procedures.

Self-Expression. A social component where an individual is able to use a variety of styles and skills to express thoughts, feelings, and needs such as pleasure, anger, distrust, agreement, and disagreement. Creative media such as art, music, Psychodrama, Role playing, and poetry can be used to help individuals to express their feeling.

Self-Fulfilling Prophesy. The expectation by a researcher or rater that a subject will perform at a certain level based on prejudice or bias toward the group to which the subject belongs.

Sensorimotor Performance Components. Individual's ability to receive sensory perceptual organization and transmit neuromusculoskeletal and motor information. The sensory domain includes Sensory awareness, and Sensory processing of Tactile, Proprioceptive, Vestibular, Visual, Auditory, Gustatory, and Olfactory information. The perceptual domain includes organizing Stereognosis, Kinesthesia, Pain response, Body scheme, Right-left discrimination, Form constancy, Position in space, Visual closure, Figure ground, Depth perception, Spatial relations, and Topographical orientation. The neuromusculoskeletal domain includes movements related to Reflexes and reactions, Range of motion, Muscle tone, Strength, Endurance, Postural control, Postural alignment, and Soft-tissue integration. The motor domain includes gross (motor) coordination, crossing the Midline, Laterality, Bilateral integration, Motor control, Praxis, Fine motor coordination/dexterity, Visual motor integration, and Oral motor control.

Sensory Awareness. Awareness of and differentiation of stimuli that are received through the sensory channels such as Auditory, Visual, Tactile, Olfactory, Gustatory, Vestibular, and Proprioceptive.

Sensory Defensiveness. An alternate term for Hypersensitivity. Persons with this condition find touch uncomfortable or irritating. Treatment that may help increase the patient's tolerance to touch is called Desensitization. See Sensory deficits and Hypersensitivity for further discussion and treatment.

Sensory Deficits. An impairment in a patient's sensory system can hinder function even though the patient may have normal motor or cognitive ability. A patient may demonstrate difficulty with sensing where the extremities are or telling that the hand is holding onto an object. A patient with decreased sensation is especially at risk for injury to the affected body part, since the patient will not be

Sensory Deficits

Sensory Deficits. *(continued)*
able to tell if the part has been placed on a dangerously sharp or hot object. Deficits may be displayed in the following sensory areas: <u>Touch awareness</u>, <u>Tactile attention</u>, <u>Touch localization</u>, <u>Touch/pressure threshold</u>, <u>Sharp/dull awareness</u>, <u>Temperature</u>, <u>Vibration awareness</u>, <u>Proprioception</u>, <u>Stereognosis</u>, and <u>Two-point discrimination</u>.

Approaches

- **Sensory Reeducation** is used with patients who demonstrate impaired, rather than absent, sensation. Patients are instructed to reinterpret stimuli within a new framework to decipher what the new stimuli mean. For example, following a stroke, a patient may state that warm water feels different than it did previous to the stroke. The patient learns what the new sensation in warm water feels like opposed to the new sensation in cold water. The patient can then learn to use these new signals or stimuli to tell the difference between the temperatures of water, even though the temperature does not feel the same as it did previously.

- **Desensitization** may be used with patients who demonstrate <u>Hypersensitivity</u> to sensory stimuli. A patient who is hypersensitive may find certain sensations uncomfortable following an injury. For example, a patient who has <u>Cubital tunnel syndrome</u> may find massage to the affected elbow very uncomfortable, while the same patient has no discomfort when the unaffected elbow is massaged. Likewise, a patient who has had a crushing injury may find a shirt sleeve to be very irritating to the affected area, even though the wound is completely healed. Desensitization is the process of presenting increasingly noxious stimuli to a patient's affected area to help increase the patient's tolerance to sensory stimulation.

- **Compensation** should be taught to patients who demonstrate absent sensation. A patient who is unable

Sensory Deficits

to feel when an affected extremity is in danger may further damage the extremity. To avoid further injury, the patient should be educated on the following principles. Sustained pressure on bony prominences will result in decreased circulation to the area. An area of low circulation is at risk of tissue damage or a sore. A sore that results from static positions is called a Decubitus ulcer, and patients should be taught to reposition themselves in bed or a wheelchair as well as to protect vulnerable areas such as the elbows or heels. Pressure may also result from splint straps that do not displace pressure over a large enough surface area. A therapist should be cautious when fabricating a splint for a patient with no sensation in the affected upper extremity. Splints may also cause pressure areas which the patient is not able to feel. The patient should be instructed to remove the splint for 15 minutes every 1–2 hours after first receiving the splint, to check for red areas that persist longer than 15 minutes. The therapist should be notified of problem areas and make adjustments as needed. Temperature can also present danger to the affected extremity. The patient should use good oven mitts/potholders and wooden or plastic utensils when cooking, good mittens if the temperature is cold outside, and thermometers to test the temperature of water, depending on the activity, if more than one extremity is affected. A patient with absent sensation will also not be able to tell if repetitive motions are causing pain to the extremity. Instruction should be provided on repetitive motion injuries and methods to reduce repetitive motion if necessary. A final danger includes the use of an infected extremity, which may cause spread of the infection. The patient should be instructed to allow an infected extremity to rest until sufficient healing has occurred. Finally, the patient should learn to use other senses to compensate for the extremity such as vision, smell, or tactile.

General Treatment Considerations

- If sensory reeducation is going to be taught, it is essential that a patient has normal cognitive ability to understand new concepts and the motivation to follow through with the training.

- Treatment should be graded so a patient can demonstrate success. If activities are too difficult, the patient will become frustrated and may want to discontinue therapy.

- The therapist should monitor treatment to prevent a patient from accidentally injuring him- or herself on sharp objects.

- Treatment usually begins with a specific activity, but it should be generalized to situations that the patient normally encounters. For example, when working on stereognosis, a patient may place the hands in a sheltered area to identify objects through tactile input from a list provided by the therapist. A patient does not usually have the convenience of a list to choose from in situations outside of the clinic. The patient should eventually work toward identifying items in a purse without looking and with no cues provided, because this more accurately resembles a real-life situation when stereognosis is used.

- The treatment environment should be free from distractions since these tasks require concentration.

- Tasks should be only 10–15 minutes in length, but the patient should participate in 2–4 sessions per day for optimal benefit.

- Most specific deficits stem from a patient's inability to sense tactile input; therefore, treatment should begin with the techniques listed under touch (or tactile) awareness. After the patient is able to perceive tactile input, more specific input such as tactile attention, touch localization, touch/pressure threshold, temperature, etc. may be practiced. The therapist should take careful note of correct and incorrect responses to document progress.

Treatment of Specific Deficits
Touch Awareness

- The therapist should provide tactile input during treatment when possible. While the patient completes ROM or strengthening tasks, the therapist can lightly stroke the affected extremity.
- Lotion may be applied to the affected extremity.
- Different textures may be rubbed against the affected area. Some textures that can be used include a terry cloth towel, cotton ball, sandpaper, moleskin, foam, leather, eraser, clay, and a feather.
- A patient can trace shapes with the finger on carpeting.
- Clay can be made into shapes.
- The patient can wash clothes by hand.
- Vibration or electric stimulation can be applied to the affected area.
- Special textures can be applied to grooming or feeding equipment to increase input.
- The patient can press out pizza dough or knead bread dough.

Touch Localization

- A patient must be able to sense tactile input before localization of the input is possible. See Touch awareness above for methods to improve tactile awareness. Treatment can then proceed with the patient practicing localization of tactile input. The therapist should record the patient's correct and incorrect responses (measurement from touched point to identified point) to document progress.

Proprioception

- Weightbearing may help increase a patient's awareness of the position of extremities.

Stereognosis

- Treatment begins while allowing the patient to use other senses such as sight or hearing to compensate for tactile impairment; but the patient should progress toward identification of objects through tactile input only. The patient can first learn to identify if objects are similar or different. The patient then learns to describe the ways in which the objects are different such as in size or shape.

- Treatment should progress from larger traits and differences to finer details.
- A patient can learn to identify objects that are placed in the hand, but the patient should progress to locating the object among various objects on the table.
- Objects that are three-dimensional are easier to identify than those that are two-dimensional, so treatment should also proceed according to this rule.
- The patient can practice locating small objects in a bowl of rice, sand, macaroni, and popcorn.
- Many small objects can be placed in a container, and the patient then removes the objects and counts them.

Hypersensitivity

- A protective device may be placed over the affected extremity, but use of the device should be gradually discontinued as treatment proceeds.
- A patient should progress through the Downey Hand Center's hierarchy of textures. The patient should then choose a texture which is tolerable and apply the texture to the affected extremity or area for 10 minutes 3–4 times a day. The hierarchy is listed in order of least noxious to most noxious. For each level, a texture is first listed which can be applied to a dowel and stroked over the affected area, and then a texture is listed which a patient can place in a container for immersion of the affected area.
  - Moleskin / Cotton
  - Felt / Terry cloth pieces
  - Closed cell foam (Quickstick) / Dry rice
  - Velvet / Popcorn

- Semi-rough cloth / Pinto beans
- Velcro loop / Macaroni
- Hard T-foam / Plastic wire insulation pieces
- Burlap / Small BB's or buckshot
- Rug back / Large BB's or buckshot
- Velcro hook / Plastic squares
- Other mediums or activities that can be used with a hypersensitive area include the following: weightbearing, massage, an Isotoner glove, TENS, Fluidotherapy, or any activity which requires use of the affected extremity or area.

Sensory Integration (SI) Therapy. An occupational therapy Frame of reference that is based on developmental, neurological, and perceptual concepts. Treatment includes various types of sensory input to help the brain to learn to organize this input for accomplishing functional activities such as Self-care and academic learning. SI has been successfully applied to individuals with Cerebral palsy, Autism, Learning disabilities, Mental retardation, Traumatic brain injury, developmental delay, and Schizophrenia. An important component of treatment is to allow the client to collaborate with the therapist in selecting activities. Vestibular stimulation, balance exercises, visual spatial awareness, motor planning, tactile exercises, and bilateral motor coordination activities are specific techniques used in treatment (Ayres, 1972). Some of the equipment used with children include swings, bolsters, slides, large balls, mattresses filled with water and foam, scooter boards, inner tubes, flash cards and sand. During treatment sessions the therapist integrates various media to stimulate the client and induce positive movements in a supportive environment. The family plays an important role in reinforcing the activities in the home.

Sensory Processing. The operation of interpreting sensory stimuli so that it is meaningful to an individual. For example, interpreting visual stimuli that are words on a

Sensory Processing. *(continued)*

sensory level without reading or understanding the words. Giving meaning to the words is a perceptual and cognitive process.

Sensory Reeducation. A method used with patients who demonstrate impaired, rather than absent, sensation. Patients are instructed to reinterpret stimuli within a new framework to decipher what the new stimuli mean. See <u>Sensory deficits</u> for further discussion and treatment.

Sequencing. The cognitive skill that involves placing information, concepts, and actions in a logical order. It is a critical skill that is related to motor planning tasks such as in dressing, in language (e.g., in telling a story), or in non-verbal communication when listening (e.g., using eye contact).

Serial Casting. A process of casting a spastic limb in its full available ROM for a prolonged period of time to provide the spastic muscles with prolonged stretch. Some research has shown that a prolonged stretch may decrease spasticity and increase ROM. The therapist fabricates a cast at full stretch of the spastic muscles. The cast is then applied for up to 3 months with removal twice daily for exercises/movement and cleansing of the skin on the affected arm. At that point, the therapist fabricates a new cast at a greater degree of stretch than the previous cast. Precautions include increased pain or skin breakdown, and the therapist should carefully monitor the condition of the patient's extremity during serial casting.

Serotonin. A neurotransmitter that occurs naturally in the brain. It plays an important role in mood behavior and sleep-wake cycle. The regulation of serotonin is important in treating <u>Depression</u>.

Sharp/Dull Awareness. The ability to discriminate between sharp and dull stimuli. This is one of many components included in a sensory evaluation to test for deficits. See <u>Sensory deficits</u> for further discussion and treatment.

Sheltered Workshop.   A supportive employment environ-ment where individuals with disabilities produce a saleable product such as in assembly work or provide a service such as lawn maintenance. Individuals are usually paid on the basis of their productivity, which can be below or at compa-rable wages for the job performed. The work can be transi-tional to competitive employment or long term. Work adjust-ment training is usually incorporated into the program.

Side-Effects of Medications.   Adverse effects in an individual that accompany the actions of a drug, such as nausea, headaches, dizziness, hypertension, dryness of mouth, blurred vision, insomnia, and tardive dyskinesia. Side effects occur because most medications have multiple effects on the body.

Signs.   Objective findings of a disease or disorder that are observed by the clinician or measured objectively through a test. Psychiatric signs can be gathered through laboratory findings indicating brain lesions, through electroencephalo-grams indicating epilepsy, or through objective tests such as *Minnesota Multiphasic Personality Inventory*.

Sling.   A fabric orthosis that fits around the upper extremity to help resist the downward pull of gravity on the head of the humerus when supporting scapula muscles are weak. Slings have often been used with patients who have hemi-plegia to presumably help maintain the position the head of the humerus in the glenoid fossa when the patient is at risk for <u>Subluxation</u>. They are most often applied for treatment when the patient is standing upright, to resist the pull of gravity and help prevent further subluxation. The use of slings has been controversial. The <u>Universal hemiplegic sling</u> does relieve the shoulder from carrying the full weight of the affected arm; however, this sling does *not* help

Sling. *(continued)*

approximate the head of the humerus. A special sling for patients with hemiplegia has a cuff that attaches around the proximal humerus. This type of sling may assist with Approximation while allowing the forearm and hand to remain free to complete movement. Slings do not cure a subluxation, and neither do they completely prevent further dislocation. When a sling passively positions the upper extremity, the muscles that need to position the humerus are not being asked to work. This may cause the supporting muscles to weaken and contribute to further subluxation. Slings are often used to help prevent pain; however subluxation itself may not be painful. A sling can sometimes increase the risk of pain because immobilization may lead to Shoulder-hand syndrome. Finally, some slings (including the universal hemiplegic sling) position the affected upper extremity in the Typical upper extremity posture seen in patients with Hemiplegia rather than attempting to disrupt the components of synergy which are acting on the extremity. Slings should be used cautiously and intermittently, while treatment should focus on the reactivation of the shoulder musculature which supports the head of the humerus in the glenoid fossa. See Orthosis.

SOAP Note. An organized method of recording a patient's progress. SOAP stands for

- *S*ubjective findings which are the reported symptoms of the patient
- *O*bjective findings of the therapist
- *A*ssessment, which is the documented analysis and summary of the findings
- *P*lan, which are the recommended treatments, therapeutic interventions, and further diagnostic tests, if necessary.

Social Conduct. Refers to eye contact, social interaction, nonverbal communication, social skills, manners, and self-expression. Social skills training are used by occupational therapists in Psychosocial rehabilitation programs to improve or develop social conduct.

Social Skills. Skills in attending/listening, conversational, supportive, problem solving, and self-control. These skills include both verbal and nonverbal behaviors. There are usually four steps in teaching any social skill:

- Psychoeducational instruction where the therapist presents information to the client regarding coping strategies and information in preventing recurrence of symptoms. Films, handouts, and homework reinforce what is learned.
- Demonstration and modeling of social skills through Role playing and Behavioral rehearsal where the therapist performs the skill. Video taping is frequently used.
- Guided practice where the therapist observes the client as he or she performs a social skill in a supportive Group therapy format and receives feedback and constructive criticism.
- Independent activities where the client begins to practice a social skill in the community and to report back to the therapist and group what difficulties he or she encountered.

Soft Tissue Integrity. Prevention of breakdowns in skin and to maintain health of interstitial tissues. Damage to soft tissue occurs in industry when workers handle sharp or abrasive objects during repetitive motions. Decubiti occur in patients who have prolonged pressure on skin during confinement in bed or sitting in a wheelchair. Strategies to prevent skin abrasions include protective barriers such as gloves, padding, and seat covers and strategies such as changing positions and job rotation.

Souques Finger Phenomenon. Flexion of the patient's affected shoulder may result in extension of the affected fingers. This phenomenon is not present in all patients with hemiplegia, but Brunnstrom (1970, 1996) discovered that shoulder flexion presented the optimal position if the therapist is trying to facilitate finger extension. See Motor control problems, Movement therapy of Brunnstrom.

Spasms.   Involuntary contractions of large muscle groups in the body. Spasms may result from lesions in the corticospinal or extrapyramidal tracts.

Spasticity.   An increase in Muscle tone, also referred to as Hypertonicity, in the affected extremity of a person who has Hemiplegia. High muscle tone most often follows after a patient has had a stroke and experienced Flaccidity, or low muscle tone. The patient will have difficulty completing AROM in the opposite direction of the spastic muscles (i.e., difficulty with finger extension if the finger flexors are spastic). Complaints of pain during PROM are also common, and caution should be taken when stretching tight muscles. See Motor control problems and Cerebral vascular accident (CVA) for treatment methods.

Spatial Dyscalculia.   Inability to arrange numbers spatially when performing math problems. For example, when completing subtraction, the columns are not straight, which can cause subtraction of the wrong numbers. Use of graph paper, or lined paper turned sideways, will help alleviate this difficulty.

Spatial Operations.   Cognitive ability to mentally manipulate the position of objects in various relationships. This ability entails being able to conceptualize distance between objects, as in driving a car, throwing a ball, turning an object upside down, or visualizing the movements of the planets around the sun. Using hand tools and constructing objects stimulate spatial operations.

Spatial Relations.   Perceptual process or ability to determine the position of objects in relationship to each other such as hitting a ball in baseball, playing tennis, or assembling parts in a factory. See Cognitive-perceptual deficits for further discussion and treatment.

Spherical Grasp.   See Grasp.

Spina Bifida.   A condition that results in malformation of the vertebrae and can be accompanied by protrusion of the meninges, spinal cord, or both. Deficits will vary, depending on the location and severity of the malformation.

Spinal Cord Injury.   A condition that occurs as a result from a lesion in the spinal cord. The level and location of the lesion directly affect the patient's function. Paraplegia or quadriplegia may occur as well as sensory loss to the affected areas. The cause may be from a traumatic experience or from tumors or infectious diseases.

Specific Treatments
- Maintain both <u>AROM</u> and <u>PROM</u>
- Increase muscle strength and endurance of the upper extremities
- Improve coordination and dexterity
- Manage spasticity
- Increase patient's awareness of <u>Sensory deficits</u>
- Increase endurance
- Improve mobility
- Educate patient on the condition/disease process
- Increase independence with ADLs
- Explore vocational and leisure opportunities as needed
- Assist patient with psychological adjustment to condition
- Increase patient's accessibility and safety within home and community
- Increase independence with driving

Contraindications/Precautions
- Monitor skin carefully as the patient is at great risk for pressure sores.
- Observe the patient for changes in respiration, especially if the patient is taking morphine.
- Do not overstretch joints, which can cause permanent joint damage.
- Monitor the patient for <u>Autonomic dysreflexia</u> and know the proper method for treating this condition.

Spirituality.   An individual's focus on meaning in life and connectiveness to the universe. It is the higher purposes that give meaning to life and is evident through faith and beliefs.

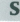

Splints.   An orthosis which is attached to a patient's body or used by the patient to help restore function. Orthoses which are applied to hands are often referred to as splints. Splints may be used to: decrease the effect of abnormal muscle tone, support a weak extremity, immobilize an extremity following surgery or trauma, or correct deformity (Coppard & Lohman, 1996).

Types of Splints
- **Static Splint**: These splints have no moving parts, so they are used for support and stability. The therapist fabricates a static splint to immobilize a joint or prevent contractures and/or deformity.
  Examples
  - Resting hand splint
  - Wrist cock-up splint
  - Ulnar deviation correction splint
  - Thumb spica splint
  - Thumb web spacer or C-bar splint
- **Dynamic Splint**. These splints have moving parts that are used to assist with proper alignment of fractures, substitute for muscles which have undergone surgical repair, increase ROM and decrease contractures, or control movement. The therapist fabricates a dynamic splint to increase mobility at a joint.
  Examples
  - Flexor tendon repair splint
  - Extensor tendon repair splint
  - Radial palsy splint
  - Extension splint for an ulnar nerve injury
- **Volar Splint**. A splint applied to the volar of the forearm, hand, and/or fingers. This type of splint may be used as a static application to immobilize the wrist, or

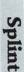

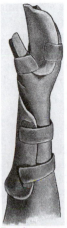

Resting
hand splint

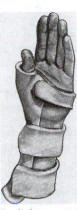

Radial gutter
thumb spica splint

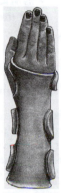

Dorsal wrist
cock-up splint

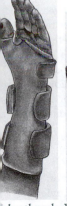

olar thumb
pica splint

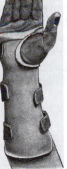

Volar wrist
cock-up splint

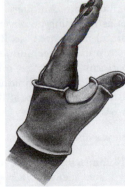

Hand based thumb
spica splint

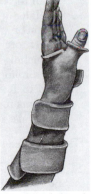

Top dorsal thumb
spica splint

as a base for hardware which will produce a dynamic application to increase ROM in the fingers.

- **Dorsal Splint**. A splint applied to the dorsal surface of the forearm, hand, and/or fingers. This type of splint may be used as a static application to immobilize the wrist without compressing the carpal tunnel, or as a base for hardware which will produce a dynamic application to substitute for extensor muscles in the case of extensor tendon repair.

Stereognosis. Ability to identify familiar objects through touch without visual cues. This is one of many components included in a sensory evaluation to test for deficits. Loss of tactile function will diminish stereognosis. See Sensory deficits for further discussion and treatment.

Stigma. Devaluation of an individual because of a disability. For example, the stigma attached to having a psychiatric disability is marked by a prejudiced attitude by a person who devalues an individual with mental illness.

Stimulation Techniques. The term used by Bobath (1978) to refer to sensory techniques used to help magnify the effect of facilitation techniques. Bobath defines facilitation techniques as Handling patterns used by the therapist to promote normal movement, so Bobath defines tapping or brushing as stimulation techniques, which are added to the handling patterns. Bobath's stimulation techniques are equal to Rood's facilitation techniques. See Motor control problems for further explanation of Bobath's approach versus Rood's approach.

STNR. See Reflexes and reactions.

Storytelling. Reminiscing about events in a person's life and recapturing visual scenes. It can also be a life review of an individual. It is used with individuals with cognitive deficits, such as Alzheimer's disease.

Stress. A term that can mean the amount of pressure on an individual (stressor) or the end result such as (stress reactions).

Stress Management. A general term that includes systematic treatment interventions to reduce the hyperarousal of the sympathetic nervous system. Biofeedback (Norris & Fahrion ,1993), Progressive relaxation, Relaxation response, meditation, Yoga, Tai-ch'i, Music therapy, Prescriptive exercise, and Cognitive-behavioral therapy are examples of techniques used in a comprehensive stress management program. In designing a stress management program the therapist should consider the following questions:

- What is the target population? Examples: individuals with Depression, arthritis, Schizophrenia, substance abuse, or Stroke.
- What are the specific goals for the group? Examples: reduce anxiety, increase the number of copers, learn relaxation methods, incorporate exercise into everyday life, or to gain insight into stressors and symptoms.
- What are the specific techniques that the client will learn? Examples: relaxation response, progressive relaxation, Biofeedback, Prescriptive exercise, nutrition, creative expression or visualization exercises.
- What will be the context for stress management? Examples: individual or Group therapy, How many sessions? How long will each session be? If group, how many clients will be in the group and where will the therapy take place?
- What modalities and therapeutic strategies will be applied? Examples: Psychoeducational with lectures and discussion, Role playing, music for relaxation, demonstrations of relaxation techniques, practice in learning techniques, learning arts and crafts, or engaging in exercises such as Tai-ch'i.
- How will the occupational therapist evaluate the effectiveness of the stress management program? Examples: Self-evaluation, standardized tests, physiological measures (Biofeedback), and clinical observation.

- What are the potential problems that reduce the effectiveness of the program? Examples: lack of client motivation, lack of compliance to stress management recommendations, and noisy or distracting environment?

Stress Reactions.   The psycho-physiological reactions in an individual that are the end results of <u>Stressors</u> minus personal resources.

Stressors.   The specific factors that precipitate a stress reaction.

Stretch.   A technique which can be used to facilitate low <u>Muscle tone</u> or inhibit high muscle tone.

- *Quick stretch* facilitates muscle tone, but the effects are temporary. The therapist stabilizes the proximal joint while quickly moving the distal joint (i.e., stabilizing the shoulder while quickly flexing the elbow to facilitate the triceps). This type of facilitation is usually applied to flexors and adductors.

- *Maintained stretch* inhibits muscle tone, according to Rood (1964); however, Rood did not suggest passive stretching. Rood's theory stated that a muscle should be positioned in its elongated state while the <u>Antagonist</u> is facilitated. This type of stretch on the <u>Agonist</u> would help lengthen the muscle's spindles and decrease the tone. A final definition of stretch is the act of applying outside forces to lengthen a muscle, as occurs during passive range of motion activities. See <u>Motor control problems</u>, <u>Rood approach</u>, and <u>Passive range of motion</u>.

Stretch Reflex.   A protective reflex which serves to limit a joint's ROM and therefore protect the muscles around the joint from being stretched too far. When a muscle is quickly stretched, the muscle spindle sends a signal to the CNS, which returns a signal that asks the muscle to contract. The strength of the contraction is often in proportion to the speed of the stretch to the muscle; however, overprotective stretch reflexes may be present in persons who demonstrate hypertonicity. See Hypertonicity.

Stroke.   See Cerebral vascular accident (CVA) for discussion and treatment

Stroking.   A technique that can either facilitate or inhibit Muscle tone. If facilitation is the desired outcome, then light stroking of 3 to 5 repetitions with 30-second rest breaks between repetitions is the technique of choice. If inhibition is the desired outcome, then slow stroking with a firm and constant pressure is applied. See Motor control problems, Rood approach for more discussion of inhibition and facilitation techniques.

Subluxation.   The process of the head of the humerus partially dislocating from the glenoid fossa as a result of abnormal tone of the supporting muscles. When the scapular muscles (specifically the Rotator cuff muscles) demonstrate low tone, the head of the humerus cannot resist the downward pull of gravity. Also, the fossa may orient backward, downward, and/or medially rather than its usual forward, upward, lateral direction, which can facilitate subluxation. If the muscles that attach to the head of the humerus become spastic, subluxation can also occur. This is demonstrated in a patient who demonstrates spasticity of the pectoral muscles accompanied by an anterior subluxation of the humerus. Treatment should focus on facilitation or inhibition of the appropriate muscles to restore orientation of the fossa and pull of the humerus into the fossa. Slings have often been used to help position the humerus into the fossa, especially while a patient with Hemiplegia stands upright and the downward pull of gravity is stronger; however, the effectiveness of slings has been questioned. See Sling.

Substance Abuse.   A psychiatric disorder in which an individual becomes dependent on a chemical substance

Substance Abuse. *(continued)*
such as alcohol, sedatives, hypnotics, anxiolytics, amphetamines, cocaine, opium, or heroin. Effects of substance abuse include delirium, psychosis, and cognitive mood disorders, sleep and eating disturbances, anxiety, and a general interference with functional activities of living. Occupational therapy treatment goals for individuals with substance abuse include <u>Social skills</u> training, vocational readiness, anger and <u>Stress management</u>, development of <u>Leisure</u> activities, self-regulation of addictive behavior, and effective time management. Specific media can include woodworking, horticulture, daily diaries, use of creative and expressive activities, <u>Role playing</u>, and values clarification. Group treatment using a <u>Psychoeducational</u> approach with <u>Cognitive-behavioral treatment</u> have been shown to be effective in treating individuals with substance abuse.

Substitution.   This method may be used by a patient during a <u>Manual muscle test</u> to help improve the patient's results even though the patient has a weakness/deficit in the motion being tested. When testing the prime movers responsible for a motion, the patient may use other stronger muscles to execute a movement if the prime movers are weak. A patient may also substitute body movements such as trunk rotation or lateral flexion to assist with movement such as shoulder abduction or horizontal adduction. Finally, the patient may consciously substitute for movement by inching the arm along a supportive surface. See <u>Appendix G</u> for a list of common substitutions used during MMT.

Superficial.   See <u>Anatomical position</u>.

Superior.   See <u>Anatomical position</u>.

Supination.   See <u>Anatomical position</u>.

Supine.   A term which refers to the position of a patient while the patient lies on a horizontal surface with the back and bottom touching the supporting surface.

Support Groups. Community groups that meet regularly and provide opportunities for individuals and their families and friends to discuss their problems openly. There are hundreds of support groups for almost every disability. Meeting times and places are often listed in local newspapers.

Examples

- Alliance for the Mentally Ill (AMI)
- Recovery Incorporated
- Alcoholics Anonymous (AA)
- Alzheimer's support group
- Multiple sclerosis
- Stroke
- Brain Injury Association
- Learning Disabilities of America

Lectures, educational films, and literature are also available at support group meetings.

Supported Employment. A concept first used with individuals with developmental disabilities. It includes job placement, work adjustment, advocacy, job coaching, and follow-up. The concept has been expanded to individuals with mental illness and other disabilities to include transitional employment and access to career development and training.

Supported Housing. Refers to enabling individuals to live in affordable housing by improving access to existing housing through federal subsidies or cooperative ventures. Rental units, single-family homes, or public housing can be supported housing.

Suspension Sling. An assistive device similar to the mobile arm support, the sling attaches to the edge of the seat back on the patient's affected side. A patient can use this device to help complete functional activities; however the patient will need to have stronger and more controlled movement of the upper extremity to use the sling successfully. See Assistive technology for further discussion of adaptive equipment.

Swan Neck Deformity. A digit that demonstrates hyperextension of the <u>PIP</u> joint with flexion of the <u>DIP</u> joint. This condition can result from the rupture of distal extensor tendons, dislocation, and volar plate laxity.

Symmetrical Tonic Neck Reflex (STNR). See <u>Reflexes and reactions</u>.

Symptoms. Reported changes in an individual that are subjective sensations such as pain, hearing voices, <u>Anxiety</u>, or seeing double images.

Syncope. Dizziness caused by a temporary decrease in blood pressure or blood flow to the brain.

Synergist. A muscle which assists the <u>Prime mover</u> in completing an action by preventing other muscles from interrupting the motion.

Syndrome. Refers to a group of symptoms or signs of an impairment or dysfunction. For example, Korsakoff's syndrome is characterized by delirium, hallucinations, memory disturbances, disorientation of time and space, confusion, and personality deterioration. Persian Gulf syndrome is characterized by respiratory and gastrointestinal disturbances, fatigue, muscle and joint pain, and memory impairment.

Systematic Desensitization. A technique developed by Wolpe (1990) and used in behavior therapy for eliminating phobias in which the client is exposed to anxiety-producing stimuli in gradual increments until the <u>Phobia</u> is eliminated.

Tactile Attention.   General ability to tell that the body is being touched in two different places/areas simultaneously. For example, the patient can tell that the arm and the leg are both being touched at the same time. This is one of many components included in a sensory evaluation to test for deficits. See <u>Sensory deficits</u> for further discussion and treatment.

Tactile Defensiveness.   Syndrome conceptualized by Jean Ayres (1972) and identified in the sensory integration literature in which an individual has an aversive reaction to being handled or touched. See <u>Sensory defensiveness</u>.

Tactile Sensation.   Receiving and interpreting stimuli through nerve endings for touch as light pressure on the skin, temperature awareness, pain, and vibration.

Tai Ch'i.   Ancient Chinese exercise designed to develop *ch'i* within the body. It can be used to rejuvenate, to heal and prevent illness and injuries, and also to lead to spiritual enlightenment. It is based on principles of rhythmic movements, equilibrium of body, effective breathing, and development of life forces in the body through a series of slow-moving, circular movements.

Tapping.   The act of lightly tapping or touching the belly of a muscle with the fingertips to facilitate low <u>Muscle tone</u>. The suggested frequency in the literature is 3 to 5 taps, which may be completed prior to or during the patient's attempt to voluntarily contract the muscle. See <u>Motor control problems</u>, <u>Rood approach</u> for further discussion of facilitation techniques.

Tardive Dyskinesia.   A motor disorder that is similar to symptoms occurring in <u>Parkinson's disease</u> such as slow, rhythmic involuntary movements, tremors, and muscular weakness. It can occur as a side-effect of long-term dosage of phenothiazines, which are tranquilizers used in the treatment of <u>Schizophrenia</u>.

Task Analysis.   See <u>Activity analysis</u>.

Temperature Discrimination.   Ability to discriminate between hot and cold stimuli. This is one of many components included in a sensory evaluation to test for deficits. See <u>Sensory deficits</u> for further discussion and treatment.

Tendon Repairs.   These injuries result in treatment that is very specialized according to the location of the laceration. Other references should be consulted for treatment also, depending on the type of treatment preferred by the physician. To help clarify treatment approaches, the zones of the hand have been listed below.

Flexor Zones of the Hand
- **Zone I**: The distal part of the middle phalanx, the distal interphalangeal joint, and the fingertip
- **Zone II**: The metacarpal bones, the metacarpophalangeal joint, the proximal phalanx, the proximal interphalangeal joint, and the proximal half of the middle phalanx
- **Zone III**: The area proximal to the metacarpal heads and the proximal palm of the hand to the carpal tunnel
- **Zone IV**: The carpal tunnel area
- **Zone V**: The crease at the wrist and up toward the forearm

Extensor Zones of the Hand
- **Zone I**: The distal interphalangeal joint
- **Zone II**: The middle phalanx
- **Zone III**: The proximal interphalangeal joint
- **Zone IV**: The proximal phalanx
- **Zone V**: The metacarpophalangeal joint
- **Zone VI**: The metacarpal
- **Zone VII**: The carpal bones
- **Zone VII**: The wrist and forearm

Zones of the Thumb
- **Zone I**: The interphalangeal joint
- **Zone II**: The proximal phalanx

- **Zone III**: The metacarpophalangeal joint
- **Zone IV**: The metacarpal
- **Zone V**: The carpal bones on the radial side of the hand

Repairs

- **Flexor Tendon Repairs.**
  - The therapist should fabricate a dorsal blocking splint to prevent over-extension of the affected finger, which may rupture the repair.
  - A dynamic outrigger should be placed on the strap on the volar side of the wrist to allow rubberbands to substitute for the action of the flexor tendons, while allowing the patient to actively extend the fingers within the protected range of extension in the dorsal blocking splint.
  - The wrist is usually positioned in 20°–40° of flexion, and the metacarpophalangeal joints are positioned in 35°–40° of flexion with the interphalangeal joints at 0° flexion to prevent contractures. Neither active flexion or passive extension should be completed until after six weeks following surgery, depending on the specific protocol being used.
  - At that time dynamic splinting may or may not be discontinued, tendon gliding exercises may begin, and mild resistance can begin between 6–8 weeks after surgery.
  - Generally, the patient may begin normal activity with the affected hand at or near 12 weeks after surgery.
  - Please refer to specific protocols for more detailed treatment of specific tendons and zones where those tendons have been lacerated.
- **Extensor Tendon Repairs.**
  - Injuries to Zones IV–VII usually result in immobilization for 3–4 weeks.
  - For injuries to Zones V–VII, the therapist will need to fabricate a dorsal-based splint which places the wrist in 40°–45° of extension.

Tendon Repairs

- A dynamic outrigger should hold the metacarpopha-langeal and interphalangeal joints in 0° extension. A stop may be placed on the outrigger to allow the patient to actively flex the fingers within a safe range to avoid rupture of the repaired tendons. Again the patient allows the outrigger or rubberbands to extend the fingers rather than actively using the extensor tendons.
- Mild strengthening may begin between 6–8 weeks after surgery
- Normal activity resuming at 10–12 weeks after surgery.
- Please refer to specific protocols for more detailed treatment of specific tendons and zones where those tendons have been lacerated.

Tendon Transfers. This is not an injury, but a surgery that is completed following an injury. Once the physician knows that nerve or muscle damage is permanent, the physician may choose to transfer a tendon from a working muscle to a bone or joint that is not able to move due to an injury. This allows the working muscle to now move the affected joint. Once surgery has been completed, the affected part should be immobilized for 3–4 weeks if the transferred tendon is a flexor tendon. Immobilization may be necessary for 4–6 weeks if the transferred tendon is a weaker extensor tendon. The therapist should fabricate a splint to help protect the tendon for 2–3 more weeks, but the splint may be removed for exercise. Gentle active range of motion may be started while using Icing, compression, or elevation to help decrease Edema. The therapist should gradually increase the exercise program while adding resistance to strengthen the transferred tendon.

Tenodesis. A natural action of the hand that results from the length of the extrinsic flexor and extensor muscles of the forearm or hand. When a person flexes the wrist, the fingers naturally extend through partial ROM. When a person extends the wrist, the fingers naturally flex through partial ROM. A patient with spinal cord injury can learn to use this motion to help compensate for weak finger flexors/extensors. By voluntarily extending the wrist, the patient can learn to flex the fingers to help grasp items. Likewise, by voluntarily flexing the wrist, the patient can learn to extend the fingers to release items.

Tenolysis. Surgery that helps free a tendon from adhesion to improve tendon gliding, which will in turn improve movement at the affected joints. This procedure may be necessary if a patient has not achieved sufficient tendon gliding following a tendon repair. The physician may need to perform surgery to free the tendon from scar tissue. Therapy should begin as soon as possible following the surgery, with the patient completing Active range of motion to achieve good tendon gliding. The patient should not complete resistive activities until 6–8 weeks following surgery, as surgery usually decreases bloodflow to the tendon and results in a weaker tendon that could rupture.

TENS. See Transcutaneous electrical nerve stimulation.

Terminal Behavior. Refers to the target goal in behavior therapy such as the cessation of smoking, the reduction of temper tantrums, or elimination of Phobias.

Termination or Stopping a Physical or Mental Activity. Cognitive task that requires the individual to understand the sequence of an activity. Individuals with brain damage or severe mental retardation may have difficulty in terminating an activity and may perseverate on the same aspects of the activity. The therapist can structure the sequence of activity to eliminate perseveration.

Tertiary Prevention. Prevention of secondary problems that can result from a disability, such as preventing decubiti in individuals with Spinal cord injury.

Test Battery. A group of tests selected to comprehensively measure an individual's capacity. In Occupational Therapy, typical areas assessed include behavior, vocational and Leisure interests, aptitudes, Self-care, and Work capacity.

Theory. A comprehensive conceptual framework that attempts to explain, for example, how individuals contract and resist disease, learn motor tasks, and develop cognitive and language functions.

Therapeutic Community. A term first coined by Maxwell Jones (1953) to describe a treatment environment created in psychiatric hospitals or community mental health centers where community meetings of staff, patients, and family are held, patient government is encouraged, and each individual takes responsibility for housekeeping tasks.

Therapeutic Milieu. An environment of support where clients feel comfortable in learning and developing social, cognitive, employment, Leisure, and Self-care skills while feeling empowered to change behavior.

Therapeutic Social Clubs. Client-centered groups where individuals can socialize, and engage in recreational activities. They can be incorporated in hospitals or in the community as drop-in centers. Beard at Fountain House in New York City was an innovator in developing therapeutic social clubs.

Therapeutic Use of Self. A term conceptualized by Jerome Frank (1958), a psychotherapist. It refers to a therapist using his or her personal behavior and feeling in providing feedback to the client.

Three-Jaw Chuck Pinch. A prehension pattern involving the thumb and first two digits. See Palmar prehension.

Time Management. Involves planning and participating in a balance of Self-care, Work, Leisure, and rest, to promote satisfaction and health. Healthy time management is related to wellness and a balance in an individual's life such as 8 hours work, 8 hours sleep, and 8 hours of <u>Self-care</u> and <u>Leisure</u>. Occupational therapists can help clients to establish priorities and to schedule activities that reduce <u>Stressors</u> to the therapist-client relationship.

Tip Prehension.   A pattern that combines opposition and flexion of the IP joint of the thumb with <u>PIP</u> and <u>DIP</u> flexion of the index finger so that the tips of the distal phalanxes are touching. This pattern is used when picking up a very small object such as a hairpin or penny.

Toileting.   An activity of daily living (ADL) essential to an individual's self-care. See <u>Self-care</u> for specific adaptive techniques, <u>Assistive technology</u> for adaptive equipment, and specific diagnoses/conditions for further discussion and treatment.

Token Economy.   A technique of behavior therapy in which clients earn tokens for specific positive behaviors or mastery of skills. Token economies have been used in psychiatric hospitals and residential schools. Tokens can be exchanged for desired foods or privileges.

Tonic Labyrinthine Reflex.   See <u>Reflexes and reactions</u>.

Tonic Lumbar Reflex.   See <u>Reflexes and reactions</u>.

Tonic Neck Reflex.   See <u>Reflexes and reactions</u>.

Topographical Orientation.   The perceptual ability to move from one location to another without assistance. This ability is enhanced by our awareness of directionality, memory of places, and spatial relations, for example, moving from one department to another within a hospital, or from one geographical location to another within a city or state. See <u>Cognitive-perceptual deficits</u> for further discussion and treatment.

Total Active Motion (TAM).   A measurement used to help record the motion of the MPs, PIPs, and DIPs due to tendon excursion. To find this number, the therapist measures active flexion and extension at each joint of a digit. The number of degrees of flexion available at each joint is added together, and the number of degrees that each joint lacks from 0° is subtracted from that sum. For example, the therapist measures the patient's joints as follows: MP = 90° flexion and lacking 5° extension (−5°); PIP = 105° flexion and lacking 15° extension (−15°); DIP = 40° flexion and full extension. To find the TAM of the digit, the therapist should add 90° + 105° + 40° − 5° − 15° = 215°. The digit should be measured while the patient makes a fist; the patient should not attempt to flex only the digit being measured. The TAM is then compared to the TAM of the corresponding finger on the opposite hand.

Total Passive Motion (TPM).   A measurement used to help record the motion of the MPs, PIPs, and DIPs which is due to joint mobility. The method for measurement and comparison is similar to TAM; the only difference is that passive motion rather than active motion is measured. See Total active motion (TAM) for method, comparison, and computation instructions.

Touch Awareness.   The ability to tell that someone or something is touching the body. This is one of many components included in a sensory evaluation to test for deficits. See Sensory deficits for further discussion and treatment.

Touch Localization.   The ability to identify the approximate area where the body is touched without visual cues. This is one of many components included in a sensory evaluation to test for deficits. See Sensory deficits for further discussion and treatment.

Touch/Pressure Threshold.   The amount of touch or pressure needed so that a patient is able to sense the stimuli. This is one of many components included in a sensory evaluation to test for deficits. See <u>Sensory deficits</u> for further discussion and treatment.

Traction.   A separation of joint surfaces that facilitates joint receptors and promotes movement, used by Voss (1967) within the framework of PNF. This technique may decrease pain or increase range of motion during treatment. See <u>Motor control problems</u>, <u>Proprioceptive neuromuscular facilitation</u> for more techniques.

Transactional analysis (TA).   A <u>Psychotherapy</u> technique developed by Berne (1961) that analyzes the roles that individuals assume in interpersonal relationships such as parent (superego), child (id), or adult (ego).

Transcutaneous electrical nerve stimulation (TENS).   A noninvasive physical agent modality which uses electrical current to help decrease pain, based on the endorphin release principle and on the gate-control theory principle. It consists of a small battery-operated unit that sends mild electrical current through the skin that interferes with transmission of painful stimuli. It is usually placed near the site of the pain such as in the lower back. Precautions are noted in using TENS include skin irritations and interfering with pacemaker. See <u>Physical agent modalities</u> for further discussion and treatment.

Transdisciplinary Team.   Professionals from various disciplines who share their roles with one another. For example, an occupational therapist may use <u>Family therapy</u> or behavior management techniques in treatment sessions after consulting with the social worker or behavioral psychologist about the procedures.

Transfers/Mobility.   An <u>Activity of daily living (ADL)</u> that is essential to an individual's self-care. See <u>Self-care</u> for specific adaptive techniques, <u>Assistive technology</u> for adaptive equipment, and specific diagnoses/conditions for further discussion and treatment.

Traumatic Brain Injury.   An insult to the brain resulting from an external object. The movement of the brain within the skull damages brain tissue. Injury occurs at the point of impact and the counter-coup. The cause of TBI is often a car accident or gunshot wound.

Specific Treatments
- Increase response to stimuli and environment
- Improve patient's positioning
- Maintain PROM
- Improve swallowing
- Increase independence with ADLs
- Improve cognitive functions
- Improve perceptual functions
- Improve visual tracking and scanning
- Improve tactile sensation and teach safety in regards to sensory loss
- Teach <u>Pain management</u>
- Teach <u>Stress management</u>
- Increase voluntary movement of the affected upper extremity
- Increase muscle strength
- Improve coordination
- Increase endurance
- Assist patient with psychological adjustment to condition
- Educate patient on condition/disease process
- Increase patient's accessibility and safety within the home and community
- Explore vocational opportunities as needed
- Assist patient in finding leisure activities

Contraindications/Precautions
- Monitor the skin for breakdown if splints are used.
- Expect plateaus during treatment, as the patient's progression can vary from one day to another.
- Be aware of the patient's medications and their side effects. Also be prepared for seizures.

- When a patient is going through an agitated stage, do not overly frustrate the patient.

Tremor.   A rhythmic contraction of opposing muscles that results in small involuntary movements at a joint.

Types of Tremors

- **Resting Tremor**: Small involuntary rhythmic movements at one or more joints that occur while the patient rests. When the patient completes voluntary movement, the movement is smooth and the small rhythmic involuntary movements disappear. Once the voluntary movement is complete, the involuntary oscillations reappear. A lesion in the basal ganglia may result in this deficit. Patients who have Parkinson's disease often display resting tremors, which occur in a pill-rolling motion. See Parkinson's disease for treatment and further discussion.
- **Intention Tremor**: A patient with this deficit demonstrates small involuntary rhythmic movements at one or more joints when attempting voluntary movement. While the patient is at rest, tremors will decrease or may disappear. Once the patient attempts movement, tremors will reappear and may hinder the patient's ability to complete the desired tasks. This deficit results from a cerebellar lesion, and patients who have multiple sclerosis often demonstrate intention tremors. See Multiple sclerosis for treatment and further discussion.

Turner's syndrome.   A congenital condition that results from only 45 chromosomes with only a single X sex chromosome. Symptoms include dwarfism, valgus of elbows, webbed neck, amenorrhea, and immature sexual development.

Two-Point Discrimination.   The ability to sense two different stimuli touching the patient on the same body part, and the threshold (or farthest distance apart) at which the two separate stimuli feel like only one stimulus. For example, the therapist may test the patient's hand to see

Two-Point Discrimination. *(continued)*

how far apart two pin points must be apart before the patient can feel that he or she is receiving two separate stimuli simultaneously. This is one of many components included in a sensory evaluation to test for deficits. See Sensory deficits for further discussion and treatment.

Typical Upper Extremity Posturing. A position mainly observed in a patient with hemiplegia who is beginning to develop Spasticity. Often, the patient will begin developing both the Flexor and Extensor synergies simultaneously; however, only one motion can be demonstrated at a time. The strongest components from each of the synergies "wins." so the patient demonstrates a pattern that includes both flexor and extensor motions. The typical motions observed are shoulder adduction and internal rotation, elbow flexion, forearm pronation, and wrist and finger flexion. See Motor control problems, Movement therapy of Brunnstrom for further discussion of synergies and treatment.

Ultrasound.   A physical agent modality that uses conversion of sound waves to heat deeper physiological tissue. Ultrasound can also be used in a nonthermal way to help drive topical medication into deeper tissue; this is called phonophoresis. See Physical agent modalities for further discussion and treatment.

Uniform Terminology.   A document of AOTA first published in 1979 (AOTA, 1994). The third edition was approved in 1994. The purpose of the document is to create a common terminology that can be used by occupational therapists in education, treatment, and documentation of practice. The document includes Performance areas, Performance components, and Performance contexts.

Unilateral Neglect.   The inability to sense or perceive stimuli presented on the side of the patient's body which is contralateral to the site of the brain lesion. This perceptual deficit may be demonstrated by the patient who has had a right CVA and does not dress the hemiplegic left arm or turn toward the left to look for food on the left side of the plate. This deficit differs from homonymous hemianopsia. A patient with neglect does not *understand* that the affected side exists, while the patient with homonymous hemianopsia simply cannot *see* the affected side. See Cognitive-perceptual deficits for further discussion and treatment.

Universal Hemiplegic Sling.   A sling often used by a patient with Hemiplegia who has a flaccid or weak upper extremity for the purpose of preventing subluxation. The sling usually has a fabric piece that fits around the affected arm from the elbow to the hand. This fabric is attached to a strap, which is fastened from the fabric near the elbow, around the patient's back and/or neck, to the fabric near the patient's wrist/hand. The strap may need to be padded with a wider thicker pad to provide more surface area and help displace pressure from the weight of the arm in the sling. The use of slings is very controversial. If Subluxation has

Universal Hemiplegic Sling. *(continued)*
already occurred, this type of sling does not help approximate the head of the humerus into the glenoid fossa; however, the sling could benefit the patient by relieving stress
on the shoulder from the weight of the entire arm. Also, a
patient who is beginning to demonstrate return of muscle
tone and movement in the affected extremity will not be
able to use the arm while it is positioned in the sling. Neurodevelopmental treatment views the use of slings as a risk
as immobilization may lead to Shoulder-hand syndrome.
This treatment theory also dislikes slings (including the universal hemiplegic sling) as they position the affected upper
extremity in the Typical upper extremity posture seen in
patients with hemiplegia, rather than attempting to disrupt
the components of synergy which are acting on the extremity. Slings should be used cautiously and intermittently,
while treatment should focus on the reactivation of the
shoulder musculature which supports the head of the
humerus in the glenoid fossa. See Slings.

Universal Precautions. Written guidelines established by
OSHA to protect health care workers who are exposed to
contagious diseases that produce blood-bourne pathogens,
such as HIV and hepatitis. Methods of control include protective clothing, puncture-resistant containers, and washing
of hands after contact with infectious materials.

Upper Motor Neuron Disorders. Lesions of the central nervous system may cause a disruption of the cell bod-
ies or axons in the tracts of the brain and spinal cord that
run to the lower motor neurons. These are referred to as
upper motor neuron lesions, and they result in increased
muscle tone or spasticity, hyperreflexia or increased Deep
tendon reflexes, clonus, and pathological reflexes. Disorders and diseases that may result in an upper motor lesion
include: stroke, Cerebral palsy, Multiple sclerosis, meningi-
tis, AIDS, syringomyelia, Traumatic brain injury, Spinal
cord injury, Amyotrophic lateral sclerosis, and Spina bifida.

Valgus.   An orthopedic term that refers to the outward bending or twisting of a body part away from the midline of the body; usually referring to the lower extremities. A similar, more common term which is often used is bowlegged.

Values.   Psychological components that include an individual's belief systems regarding ethics, moral behavior, standards of conduct, tolerance for others, occupational choices, and cultural morés. Values are formed by family, cultural influences, peers, and religious beliefs. Group activities such as Values clarification exercises can be helpful in clarifying and shaping an individual's values and beliefs.

Values Clarification.   "An intervention approach that utilizes a form of questioning and a set of activities or strategies to help individuals learn the valuing process" (Franklin, 1986, p. 41). This process helps an individual to choose, affirm, and act on one's beliefs.

Varus.   An orthopedic term that refers to the inward bending or twisting of a body part toward the midline of the body; usually refers to the lower extremities. A similar, more common term which is often used is knock-kneed.

Verbal Cues.   Directions given prior to movement or feedback from the therapist during movement to assist the patient in completing a desired motion correctly. This term was a technique used by Voss (1967) to help the patient reach the goal of movement during treatment. See Motor control problems, Proprioceptive neuromuscular facilitation for more techniques.

Vestibular Sensation.   Receiving and interpreting stimuli from the receptors of the inner ear in regard to the position and movement of the head. It is influenced by gravitational factors and affects balance while moving. For example, an individual with a vestibular dysfunction could experience dizziness and have a staggered walk.

Vestibular Stimulation. Stimulation of the vestibular system, which controls equilibrium and reactions to gravity. Sensory integrative therapists use vestibular stimulation in treatment by using swings, hassocks, therapy balls, and scooter boards.

Vibration. A facilitation technique that helps increase low Muscle tone. An electrical vibrator, which has a high speed of vibration per second, is the most effective tool for this technique. The vibration should be applied to the muscle belly which is slightly stretched, and it should be applied parallel to the muscle fibers for 1–2 minutes. The effects of this method are present only while the vibration is being applied. See Motor control problems, Rood approach for further discussion of facilitation techniques.

Vibration Awareness. The ability to sense vibration. This is one of many components included in a sensory evaluation to test for deficits. See Sensory deficits for further discussion and treatment.

Visual Acuity. The ability to focus on objects both at near and far distances. Visual acuity, Visual fields, and Oculomotor function comprise the Visual foundation skills which may decrease perception or negatively affect a test of perception. See Cognitive-perceptual deficits for further discussion and treatment of perceptual problems.

Visual Closure. The perceptual process of identifying a form or word from an incomplete presentation. Reading is an example of visual closure when individuals scan words quickly.

Visual Cues. Cues that assist a patient in understanding the desired movement. Demonstration of the desired movement by the therapist or positioning of an activity or the therapist in the place where movement is supposed to end. This term was a technique used by Voss (1967) to help the patient identify the goal of movement during treatment.

See Motor control problems, Proprioceptive neuromuscular facilitation for more techniques.

Visual Fields.   A person with intact visual fields must be able to see objects in each of the four quadrants of vision with each eye. Visual fields, Visual acuity, and Oculomotor function comprise the Visual foundation skills that may decrease perception or negatively affect a test of perception. See Cognitive-perceptual deficits for further discussion and treatment of perceptual problems.

Visual Foundation Skills.   These skills are comprised of Visual acuity, Visual fields, and Oculomotor function. A person with impaired visual foundation skills may demonstrate either decreased perception or a poor score on a test of perception (even though some perceptual skills can be functional without vision, such as right/left discrimination). See Cognitive-perceptual deficits for further discussion and treatment of perceptual problems.

Visual Sensation.   Receiving and interpreting stimuli through the eyes such as form, color, and pattern. Damage to visual sensation includes *myopia* (near sightedness), *presbyopia* (farsightedness), *strabismus* (crossed-eyes), *stigmatism* (inability to focus clearly), *hemianopia* (blindness in one half of the visual field), and *nystagmus* (involuntary movements of the eyeball).

Visualization.   Imagining the working's of one's own body or inner experiences to encourage healing and well-being. Visualization exercises are used in conjunction with relaxation and meditation in comprising a stress or pain management program. The steps in a visualization exercise are:
- Have the client sit in a comfortable chair with his or feet on the floor and hands in the lap.
- With the client's eyes closed, have the client create a relaxed state through meditation or the relaxation response.

- The therapist should explain to the client the purpose of the visualization exercise such as to reduce anxiety, decrease stress reactions, or facilitate sleep.
- The therapist uses a visualization tape or guides the client through the exercise such as building a dream house.

Vocational Rehabilitation. The restoration of <u>Work</u> functions in individuals with mental or physical disabilities.

Volar. A term referring to the surface of the palm or sole of the foot.

Volar Splint. See <u>Splint</u>.

Weakness.   Lack of the muscle tension necessary for maintaining posture or moving body parts through controlled and purposeful patterns to complete a task. Various conditions can lead to weakness, which may be generalized to the entire body or specifically located in one area of the body. Weakness should be treated to increase a patient's independence with functional activities as well as to prevent deformities. To increase a patient's strength, the muscle needs to recruit more motor units to fire during contraction of the muscle. This may be accomplished by applying stress to the muscle to the point of fatigue. Stress may be in the form of increased resistance to movement, velocity of movement, type of contraction, duration of exercise, or the frequency of exercise. The therapist includes this in the patient's plan of treatment as an adjunctive treatment, to help enable the patient to have sufficient strength in order to complete functional activities. Some examples of strengthening activities are listed below. See Manual muscle test for the method of testing the patient's strength to monitor progress during treatment.

Treatment Methods

- Theraband exercises: For the upper extremity, the patient should hold a stretchy piece of rubber to give resistance while completing all shoulder and elbow motions including shoulder flexion/extension, abduction/adduction, internal/external rotation, horizontal abduction/adduction, and elbow flexion/extension
- Dowel or broomstick exercises with a weight applied: Again the patient completes exercises for all motions of the shoulder and elbow
- Bilateral sander
- Beanbag activities: The patient slides the bags off a large table, to either side or forward, or tosses the bags into a bucket placed at a distance
- Skateboard with or without weights applied: The patient places the affected upper extremity on a skateboard and

moves it across the surface of a table from side to side and forward/back

- Ring tree: The patient may use one or both extremities to retrieve one ring at a time from a horizontal rod on one side of the "tree" and move it to a horizontal rod on the other side of the "tree"
- Removing items from cupboards/shelves
- Wheelchair pushups
- Dressing
- Pulleys
- Clothespins: The patient can place or remove clothespins from various heights and widths of horizontal and vertical bars
- Any activity that requires lifting the upper extremity against gravity
- Upper extremity bicycle: Most bicycles allow the therapist to adjust the tension to provide greater resistance to movement when needed
- Theraputty exercises: The patient should squeeze the putty and complete exercises to help strengthen gross grasp, wrist flexion/extension, finger flexion/extension, abduction/adduction, thumb flexion/extension, abduction/adduction, and opposition
- Resistive pegboards: The patient can place pegs into a pegboard that provides resistance to insertion and removal of the pegs
- Stirring mixtures
- Opening containers
- Drying dishes
- Lifting pans
- Sliding an object up and down an inclined surface will produce a dynamic application to increase ROM in the fingers.

Weight Bearing. A technique used by Bobath (1978) to help normalize abnormal muscle tone and increase the patient's voluntary control of movement with the involved extremity. See <u>Motor control problems</u>, <u>Neurodevelopmen-tal treatment</u> for further explanation of weightbearing

Wernicke's Aphasia.   See <u>Aphasia</u>.

Wheelchair Positioning.   A patient should be positioned in a wheelchair to decrease the risk of falling, provide safety in swallowing, prevent contractures, maintain skin integrity, reduce the use of restraints (when possible), and decrease abnormal tone or abnormal postures. See <u>Position-ing</u> for treatment.

Whirlpool.   A physical agent modality that can be classi-fied as hydrotherapy. This modality is used for many pur-poses during treatment including the heating of superficial tissue, debridement of wounds, and providing assistance or resistance to active motion. See <u>Physical agent modalities</u> for further discussion and treatment.

Williams Syndrome.   A congenital condition which results in mental retardation, a mild stunt in growth, cardio-vascular problems, and high blood calcium levels in some cases.

Work.   Paid or unpaid activity that contributes to subsistence, produces a service or product, and is culturally meaningful to the worker. Work can be driven by internal motivation if the individual engages in work purely for the inherent job satis-faction, pleasure, or self-accomplishment that results. For example, a creative artist or composer may be working to express a feeling or create a new composition without con-cern for material reward. The creative individual may spend many hours on work without pay as intrinsic motivation. On the other extreme is the individual who dislikes his or her job, such as a factory worker who works for subsistence only. This is an example of extrinsic motivation. Probably the highest level of job satisfaction is to work at a job that one enjoys and to be paid a high salary. This may be true for some profes-sional athletes or successful artists. Most individuals work to

Work. *(continued)*
support their standard of living while selecting a job that they enjoy. Some individuals engage in full-time volunteer work in activities that they find rewarding. Housewives or house husbands work at home for no monetary compensation while performing full-time work in child care, household tasks, and cooking. All of these activities are work. For the occupational therapist, evaluating the client's work and role as a worker are important aspects of treatment.

Work Hardening or Work Conditioning. An interdisciplinary team approach that applies a highly structured environment with supervised, goal oriented activities, designed to maximize the injured worker's return to work (Demers, 1992). The components of a work conditioning program include the following activities:
- Increase muscle strengthening, ROM and coordination by using purposeful and graded activities to improve function in biomechanical, neuromuscular, and cardiovascular, areas
- Intervene with psychosocial and <u>Stress management</u> programs
- Employ functional goal directed activities
- on the job work tasks using functional work capacity evaluations such as the BTE or Isenhagen
- simulated work samples
- <u>Self-care</u> activities
- body mechanic exercises
- Transition from acute treatment to return to work considering these factors:
  - What are the results of an ergonomic job assessment?
  - Would modifying the job or altering the work environment reduce risks for on the job injury?
  - Is worker able to regain, before injury, level of productivity?
  - Does worker adhere to safety rules of industry?
  - Can worker tolerate physical demands of job?
  - Is worker's behavior consistent with employee expectations?

Work Samples.   Well-defined activities that are similar to an actual job. They can be used to assess an individual's vocational aptitude, worker characteristics, and vocational interests (Nadolsky, 1974). Examples of work samples include Valpar, Micro-Tower, and McCarron-Dial.

Work Simplification.   A treatment technique that divides tasks into smaller steps or uses simple methods to make activities easier. A patient who has low endurance may require this technique to help preserve energy. A patient who has arthritis may benefit from work simplification to reduce stress on the joints. Any person with decreased strength will improve his or her ability to complete activities independently if the person uses the easiest method possible. See Energy conservation, a related topic, for techniques to preserve a patient's energy during tasks.

Self-care Tasks
- Gather necessary items before beginning each task.
- Choose light, loose-fitting clothing or clothing with elastic waistbands and cuffs. Make sure the elastic is loose enough to slip over the hips or hands.
- Use velcro closures instead of buttons, hooks, or shoelaces.
- Sit in a firm, straight-backed chair for good support when dressing.
- Fasten a brassiere at the front of the body and then turn it around to the back.
- Wear slip on shoes. Elastic shoelaces may be used to convert tie shoes into slip on shoes. A long-handled shoehorn can help a person avoid bending.
- Use belts with magnetic fasteners that require little force to fasten.
- Carry lightweight wallets or purses and eliminate all unnecessary articles from them.
- Sit while grooming whenever possible.
- Use built-up handles on grooming items to provide an easier grip.

- Shave with an electric razor rather than a hand-held razor.
- Have hair done by a professional or family member. Consider a short, easy style to maintain good appearance.
- Use a shower caddy to hold necessary items in the shower.
- Sit while undressing, showering, drying, and dressing.
- Keep baking soda in the bathroom and sprinkle some into bathwater to prevent a ring from forming around the tub. This will prevent scrubbing later.
- Use a long-handled sponge to reach feet and back.
- A terry-cloth robe will help absorb water after bathing and prevent the need for thorough drying.

Kitchen/Meal Preparation Tasks

- Plan menus before shopping.
- Plan the shopping list according to the layout of the store to eliminate extra trips.
- Shop when the store is not busy.
- Shop at a store where employees will unload the cart, bag the groceries, and carry the groceries to the car.
- Ask an employee to help lift heavy items.
- Ask an employee to bag your groceries lightly to make lifting and carrying from the car easier.
- If possible, have a family member sort and store groceries.
- Use a wheeled cart to transport groceries or take rest breaks between trips to the car for the groceries.
- Store canned goods so that the same items are lined up behind one another. This eliminates the need to remove many cans when looking for ingredients.
- Plan menus that require short preparation time and little effort. Use frozen foods, mixes, and convenience foods.
- Sit on a stool or at the table when preparing a meal.
- Use convenient appliances such as an electric can opener, food processor, or electric mixer, when possible.

- Slide items to transport them to the sink, refrigerator, or stove.
- Use a wheeled cart to carry items to the table for the meal and remove dirty dishes after the meal.
- Serve directly from the baking dish or pan used to cook the food to prevent extra dirty dishes.
- If entertaining, arrange a buffet where guests serve themselves.
- Use disposable dishes, napkins, and silverware.

Household/Cleaning Tasks

- Ask a family member make the bed for you.
- Allow space on both sides of the bed to enable the person to walk around it easily.
- Make only one trip around the bed. Begin by smoothing the sheets and blankets at the head of the bed on one side. Walk to the foot of the bed and smooth covers there. Then walk around to the other side of the bed and smooth toward the head of the bed on that side.
- Use a ping-pong paddle or yardstick to tuck in sheets.
- Eliminate knickknacks to decrease the amount of dusting.
- Use a feather duster. Sit while dusting when possible.
- Use a lightweight broom, mop, or vacuum. A self-propelled vacuum will further reduce work.
- Use a long-handled dust pan.
- Place a wastebasket in every room to eliminate trips.
- Place a pail of water for mopping on a dolly with wheels.
- Use a mop with a squeeze control on the handle.
- Store all cleaning supplies together in a bucket that can be placed on a dolly with wheels.
- Purchase a duplicate set of cleaning supplies for each story of the house.
- Ask family members for assistance with heavier cleaning tasks.

Laundry

- Use paper towels to reduce the amount of laundry.

- Have frequent wash days to avoid large loads.
- Position the laundry facilities on the main floor of the home if possible.
- Use a wheeled cart to transport dirty clothes to the laundry area.
- If the laundry facilities are in the basement, use a laundry chute.
- Sit while sorting clothes at a table.
- Place brassieres, aprons, or other fine clothing in plastic bags with holes in them or special laundry bags to avoid tangling.
- When transferring wet clothes from the washer, remove a small amount at a time.
- Purchase a laundry basket on wheels.
- Use tongs to remove articles that cannot be easily reached from the washer or dryer.
- Consider taking heavy items such as blankets or bedspreads to the laundromat for the attendants to launder.
- Sit while removing items from the dryer. Position a table on the other side of the chair, so the person can fold and sort clean laundry on the table while remaining seated.
- Avoid line drying if possible. If this is not possible, have the line within easy reach. Use push type rather than the spring type clothespins. Keep pins within easy reach also. Ask for assistance to transport clothing to the line or use a wheeled cart.
- Purchase permanent press or wrinkle-free articles of clothing.
- Do not press items that can "pass" like sleepwear, sheets, T-shirts, etc.
- Consider using a hand-held steamer unit like department stores use to get rid of wrinkles.
- Select a lightweight iron and pad the handle if needed.
- Sit while ironing. Use an adustable ironing board.
- Slide the iron rather than lifting it on and off the garment.
- Use a rack on wheels for hanger items.

- Iron in several short sessions rather than completing all the clothes at once.

Yard Work

- Take frequent rest breaks.
- Sit on a stool when working in the garden.
- Use long-handled equipment for gardening.
- Store tools together in a container and store the tools near the garden if possible.
- Consider using raised boxes for gardening.
- Ask for help from a family member or friend if the activity causes pain.
- Take advantage of power tools and labor-saving devices such as a riding or self-propelled lawn mower.

Recreation

- Use assistive technology, such as a cardholder, during activities. A clean, upturned hairbrush can also hold cards.
- Use an automatic card shuffler.
- Substitute weaving for knitting and crocheting.
- Avoid prolonged flexion of the fingers. Let a hoop hold needlework.
- Take frequent rest breaks.
- Use elastic scissors that remain open and require little pressure to close and cut items.
- Prop a book in a bookstand, or place it on a pillow on the lap.
- Lay a newspaper flat across a table.
- Use good posture while reading, playing cards, sewing, or completing other recreational activities.
- When fishing, use a rod holder to free hands during long waits.
- Use a golf cart to conserve energy for the game itself.

Work Simplification

Yoga.   As used in the Western world, an Eastern meditative discipline that has been associated almost exclusively with exercises, physical postures, and regulation of breathing. The aim is to achieve the harmony of body, mind, and spirit.

References

American Occupational Therapy Association. (AOTA). (1994). *Uniform terminology for occupational therapy: Application to practice* (3rd ed.). Rockville, MD: Author.

American Psychiatric Association. (1952). *Diagnostics and statistical manual: Mental disorders* (1st ed). Washington, DC: Author.

American Psychiatric Association. (1994.). *Diagnostic and statistical manual of psychiatric disorders* (4th ed.). Washington, DC: Author.

Anthony, W. A. (1979). *The principles of psychiatric rehabilitation.* Amherst, MA: Human Resources Press.

Atchison, B. (1995). Cardiopulmonary diseases. In C. A. Trombly (Ed.), *Occupational therapy for physical dysfunction* (4th ed., pp. 881–882). Baltimore, MD: Williams & Wilkins.

Ayres, A. J. (1972). *Sensory integration and learning disorders.* Los Angeles, CA: Western Psychological Services.

Baker, F., & Intagliata , J. (1992). Case management. In R. P. Liberman (Ed.), *Handbook of psychiatric rehabilitation* (pp. 213–243). Boston, MA: Allyn & Bacon.

Beck, A. T. (1976). *Cognitive therapy and emotional disorders.* New York, NY: International Universities Press.

Berne, E. (1961). *Transactional analysis in psychotherapy.* New York, NY: Grove.

Bobath, B. (1990). *Adult hemiplegia: Evaluation and treatment* (3rd ed.). London, England: William Heinemann Medical Books.

Brown, G. W., Birley, J. L. T., & Wing, J. K. (1972). Influence of family life on the course of schizophrenia disorder: A replication. *British Journal of Psychiatry, 121,* 241–258.

Brunnstrom, S. (1970). *Movement therapy in hemiplegia.* New York, NY: Harper & Row.

Brunnstrom, S. (1996). *Clinical kinesiology* (5th ed.). Philadelphia, PA: F. A. Davis.

Cameron, M. H. (1999). *Physical agents in rehabilitation: From research to practice.* Philadelphia, PA: Saunders

Cannon, (1932). *The wisdom of the body.* New York, NY: Norton.

Carling, P. J. (1995). *Return to community building support systems for people with psychiatric disabilities.* New York, NY: Guilford.

Carlson, N. C. (1997). Occupational therapy. In B. O'Young, M. A. Young, & S. A. Stiens (Eds.), *PM & R secrets* (pp. 139–143). Philadelphia, PA: Hanley & Belfus, Inc.

Coppard, B. M., & Lohman, H. (Eds.). (1996). *Introduction to splinting.* St. Louis, MO: Mosby.

Cummings, J. P. (1992). Additional therapeutic uses of electricity. In M. R. Gersh (Ed.), *Electrotherapy in rehabilitation* (pp. 328–340). Philadelphia, PA: F. A. Davis.

Demers, L. (1992). *Work hardening: A practical guide.* Stoneham, MA: Andover.

DeVahl, J. (1992). Neuromuscular electrical stimulation (NMES) in rehabilitation. In M. R. Gersh (Ed.), *Electrotherapy in rehabilitation* (pp. 218–268). Philadelphia, PA: F. A. Davis.

Early, M. B. (1998). *Physical dysfunction: Practice skills for the occupational therapy assistant.* St. Louis, MO: Mosby.

Ellis, A., & Whiteley, J. M. (Eds.). (1979). *Theoretical and empirical foundations of rational-emotive therapy.* Pacific Grove: CA: Brooks/Cole.

Frank, J. (1958). The therapeutic use of self. *American Journal of Occupational Therapy, 12,* 215–225.

Frankl, V. (1967). *Man's search for meaning.* Boston, MA: Beacon.

Franklin, D. (1986). A comparison of the effectiveness of Values Clarification presented as a personal computer program versus a traditional therapy group: A pilot study. *Occupational Therapy in Mental Health, 6*(3), 39–52.

Gersh, M. R. (1992). Transcutaneous electrical nerve stimulation (TENS) for management of pain and sensory pathology. In M. R. Gersh (Ed.), *Electrotherapy in rehabilitation* (pp. 149–196). Philadelphia, PA: F. A. Davis.

Glasser, W. (1965). *Reality therapy; A new approach to psychiatry.* New York, NY: Harper & Row.

Hood, C. (1959). The challenge of dance therapy. *Journal of Health, Physical Education, and Recreation, 30,* 17–18.

Hislop, H. J., Montgomery, J., & Connelly, B. (1995). *Daniel's and Worthingham's muscle testing: Techniques of manual examination* (6th ed.). Philadelphia, PA: W. B. Saunders.

Jacobson, E. (1929). *Progressive relaxation.* Chicago, IL: University of Chicago.

Jacobson, E. (1978). *You must relax* (4th ed.). New York, NY: McGraw-Hill.

Jones, M. (1953). *The therapeutic community*. New York, NY: Basic Books.

Kabat, H. (1961). Proprioceptive facilitation in therapeutic exercise. In S. Licht (Ed.), *Therapeutic exercise* (2nd ed., pp. 327–343). New Haven, CT: Elizabeth Licht.

Kendall, F. P., McCreary, E. K., & Provance, P. G. (1993). *Muscles: Testing and function* (4th ed.). Baltimore, MD: Williams & Wilkins.

Keyserling, W. M., Armstrong, T. J., & Punnett, C. (1991). Ergonomic job analysis: A structured approach for identifying risk factors associated with overexertion injuries and disorders. *Applied Occupational Environmental Hygiene, 6*, 353–363.

Kielhofner, G. (1997). *Conceptual foundations of occupational therapy* (2nd ed.). Philadelphia, PA: F. A. Davis.

Kloth, L. C. (1992). Electrotherapeutic alternative for the treatment of pain. In M. R. Gersh (Ed.), *Electrotherapy in rehabilitation* (pp. 197–215). Philadelphia, PA: F. A. Davis.

Levy, F. J. (1988). *Dance/movement therapy a healing art*. Reston, VA: The American Alliance for Health, Physical Education, Recreation, and Dance.

Michlovitz, S. L. (1990a). Biophysical principles of heating and superficial heat agents. In S. L. Michlovitz (Ed.), *Thermal agents in rehabilitation* (2nd ed., pp. 88–106). Philadelphia, PA: F. A. Davis.

Michlovitz, S. L. (1990b). Cryotherapy: The use of cold as a therapeutic agent. In S. L. Michlovitz (Ed.), *Thermal agents in rehabilitation* (2nd ed., pp. 63–85). Philadelphia, PA: F. A. Davis.

Moore, K. L. (1992). *Clinically oriented anatomy*. Baltimore, MD: Williams & Wilkins.

Nadolsky, J. M. (1974). The work sample in vocational evaluation: A consistent rationale. *Vocational Evaluation and Work Adjustment Bulletin, 7*, 2–5.

Nichols, D. S. (1996). The development of postural control. In J. Case-Smith, A. S. Allen, & P. N. Pratt (Eds.), *Occupational therapy for children* (3rd ed., pp. 247–267). St. Louis, MO: Mosby.

Norkin, C. C. & Levangie, P. K. (1992). *Joint structure and function: A comprehensive analysis* (2nd ed.). Philadelphia, PA: F. A. Davis.

Norris, P. A., & Fahrion S. L. (1993). Autogenic biofeedback in psychophysiological therapy and stress management. In P. M. Lehrer & R. L. Woolfolk (Ed.), *Principles and practices of stress management,* (2nd ed., pp. 231–262). New York, NY: Guilford.

Ottenbacher, K. J., & Cusick, A. (1989). Goal attainment scaling as a method of clinical service evaluation. *The American Journal of Occupational Therapy,* 44(6), 519–525.

Palmer, M. L., & Epler, M. E. (1998). *Fundamentals of musculoskeletal assessment techniques* (2nd ed.). Philadelphia, PA: Lippincott.

Perls, F. (1969). *Gestalt therapy verbatim.* Moab, UT: Real People Press.

Ratan, R. R. (1997). Neurologic evaluation of the rehabilitation patient. In B. O'Young, M. A. Young, & S. A. Stiens (Eds.), *PM & R secrets* (pp. 99–106). Philadelphia, PA: Hanley & Belfus, Inc.

Rogers, C. (1951). *Client-centered therapy.* Boston, MA: Houghton Mifflin.

Rolf, I. (1977). *Rolfing: The integration of human structures.* Santa Monica, CA: Dennis-Landman.

Rood, M. (1962). The use of sensory receptors to activate, facilitate and inhibit motor response, autonomic and somatic in developmental sequence. In C. Stately (Ed.), *Approaches to treatment of patients with neuromuscular dysfunction.* Third International Congress, World Federation of Occupational Therapists, Dubuque, IA: William Brown Group.

Slavson, S. R. (1943). *An introduction to group therapy.* New York, NY: The Commonwealth Fund.

Sleeve, H. (1974). *Stress without distress.* Philadelphia, PA: Lippincott.

Stein, F., & Cutler, S. K. (1998). *Psychosocial occupational therapy: A holistic approach.* San Diego: Singular Publishing Group.

Sullivan, H. S. (1963). *The fusion of psychiatry and social science.* New York, NY: W. W. Norton.

Tan, J. C. (1998). *Practical manual of physical medicine and rehabilitation: Diagnostics, therapeutics, and basic problems.* St. Louis, MO: Mosby.

Trainor, J., & Church, K. (1984). *A framework for support for people with severe mental disabilities.* Toronto, Canada: Canadian Mental Health Association

Von Bertalanffy, L. (1950). The theory of open systems in physics and biology. *Science, 111,* 23–29.

Voss, D. E. (1967). Proprioceptive neuromuscular facilitation. *American Journal of Physical Medicine, 46*(1), 838–898.

Voss, D. E., Ionta, M. K., & Myers, B. J. (1985). *Proprioceptive neuromuscular facilitation: Patterns and techniques* (3rd ed.). New York, NY: Harper & Row.

Walsh, M. T. (1990). Hydrotherapy: The use of water as a therapeutic agent. In S. L. Michlovitz (Ed.), *Thermal agents in rehabilitation* (2nd ed., pp. 109–132). Philadelphia, PA: F. A. Davis.

Wolpe, J. (1990). *The practice of behavior therapy* (4th ed.). Elmsford, NY: Persimmon.

World Health Organization (WHO). (1980). *International classification of impairments, disabilities, and handicaps* (ICIDH). Geneva, Switzerland: Author

Wykoff, W. (1993). The psychological effects of exercise on non-clinical and clinical populations of adult woman: A critical review of the literature. *Occupational Therapy in Mental Health, 12*(3), 69–106.

APPENDIX A

Commonly Used
Medical Abbreviations

/d	per day	CP	cerebral palsy
a	of each	CSF	cerebrospinal fluid
a.c.	before a meal		
ACTH	adrenocortico-tropic hormone	CVA	cerebrovascular accident
ad lib.	freely	D and C	dilatation and curettage
ADA	Americans with Disabilities Act	DIP	distal interpha-langeal
ADD	attention deficit disorder	Dx	diagnosis
ADHD	attention-deficit hyperactivity disorder	ECG	electrocardiogram
		ECT	electroconvulsive therapy
admov.	Apply	ED	emergency departure
AIDS	acquired immuno deficiency syndrome	EEG	electroencephalo-gram
ALS	amyotrophic lateral sclerosis	EMG	electromyogram
		ER	emergency room
alt.dieb	every other day	FAS	fetal alcohol syndrome
ap	before dinner		
b.i.d.	twice a day	GBS	Guillain-Barré syndrome
bib.	drink		
bol.	pill	GI	gastrointestinal
BP	blood pressure	HIV	human immuno-deficiency virus
c	with		
CBC	complete blood count	IDEA	Individuals with Disabilities Education Act of 1990
CMC	carpometacarpal joint		
CNS	central nervous system	IEP	Individualized Education Plan

IFSP	Individualized Family Service Plan		Technology Society of North America
IM	intramuscular	s(sans)	without
in d.	daily	SCI	spinal cord injury
IQ	intelligence quotient	SES	socioeconomic status
ITP	Individualized Transition Plan	STD	sexually transmitted disease
IV	intravenous		
kg	kilogram	t.i.d.	three times a day
lb	pound	TBI	traumatic brain injury
MCP	metacarpopha-langeal		
MD	muscular dystrophy		
MED	minimum effective dose		
MMR	measles-mumps-rubella vaccine		
MR	mental retardation		
MS	multiple sclerosis		
p	after		
p.c.	after meals		
PIP	proximal interphalangeal		
p.r.n.	as needed		
q.h.	every hour		
q.i.d.	four times a day		
quotid	everyday		
RBC	red blood cells		
REM	rapid eye movement		
RESNA	Rehabilitation Engineering and Assistive		

Health Organizations and World Wide Web Addresses

ABILITY	Ability Project www.ability.org.uk	AHA	American Heart Association www.amhrt.org
ABLE DATA	part of NIDRR www.abledata.com	AM	Alternative Medicine www.ability.org.uk/alternat.html
ACRM	American Congress of Rehabilitation Medicine www.acrm.org	AMA	American Medical Association www.ama-assn.org
ADA	Americans with Disabilities Act (Document Center) janweb.icdi.wvu.edu	AOTA	American Occupational Therapy Association www.aota.org
ADAPT	American Disabled for Attendant Programs Today www.adapt.org	APA	American Psychological Association www.apa.org
AF	Arthritis Foundation www.arthritis.org	APTA	American Physical Therapy Association www.apta.org
AFB	American Foundation for the Blind www.afb.org	ARC	Association for the Retarded Citizens of the US www. theArc.org

ARTSUSA	Americans for the Arts (Disabled) www.artsusa.org	DS	Down Syndrome www.nas.com/downsyn
ASHA	American Speech-Language Hearing Association www.asha.org	ES	Easter Seals www.seals.com
		JCAHO	Joint Commission on Accreditation of Healthcare Organizations www.jcaho.org
ASIA	Spinal Injuries Association www.goweb.com/sia		
Autism Resources	www.autism-resources.com	MHN	Mental Health Net www.cmhc.com
CARF	The Rehabilitation Accreditation Commission www.carf.org	NAMI	National Alliance for the Mentally Ill www.nami.org
CC	Canine Companions www.caninecompanions.org	NAOTD	National Alliance of the Disabled www.naotd.org
DHHS	Department of Health and Human Services www.os.dhhs.gov	NARIC	National Rehabilitation Information Center www.cais.com/naric
DP	Disability Page www.eskimo.com/~dempt/disability.html	NARHA	North American Riding for the Handicapped Association http://narha.org

NICHCY	National Information Center for Children and Youth with Disabilities www.nichcy.org		Health www.cdc.gov/niosh
		NRCTBI	National Resource Center for Traumatic Brain Injury www.neuro.pmr.vcu.edu
NIDRR	National Institute on Disability and Rehabilitation Research www.ed.gov/offices/OSERS/NIDRR		
		OP	Orthopedics and Prosthetics Network Connection www.psn.net/~oandpnet
NIH	National Institutes of Health www.nih.gov		
		OSEP	Office of Special Education Programs www.ed.gov/offices/OSERS/OSEP
NIMH	National Institute of Mental Health www.nimh.nib.gov		
		OSERS	Office of Special Education and Rehabilitation www.ed.gov/offices/OSERS
NINDS	National Institute of Neurological Disorders and Stroke www.ninds.nih.gov		
		OSHA	Occupational Safety and Health Administration www.osha.gov
NIOSH	National Institute for Occupational Safety and		
		RESNA	Rehabilitation Engineering and Assistive Technology

	Society of North America www.resna.org	UCP	United Cerebral Palsy www.ucp.org
RN	Rehab NET www.rehabnet.com	USDE	United States Department of Education www.ed.gov
SCIIN	Spinal Cord Injury Information Network www.spinal-cord.uab.edu	WHO	World Health Organization www.who.int
SI	Sensory Integration International http://home.earthlink.net/~sensoryint	Yahoo	Yahoo disability resources www.yahoo.com/society_and_culture/disability

APPENDIX C

Orthotics and Orthoses
Exoskeletal or External Devices
to Limit or Assist Motion in Joints of Body

Category of Device	Types	Materials	Purpose	Disability Examples
Crutch	Straight canes, forearm crutches, underarm crutches, quad canes, walkers	Wood, metal, plastic	Support or replace limb	Amputee, fracture, sprain
Splint	Static: no moving parts • Wrist cock: up splint • Resting hand splint • Ulnar deviation correction splint • Thumb web spacer	Aluminum, metal, and plastic	1. Immobilization: prevent movement 2. Correction: correct deformity 3. Preventive: contractures in muscles	Fracture Burns Arthritis Peripheral nerve injury Spinal cord injury

(continued)

(continued)

Category of Device	Types	Materials	Purpose	Disability Examples
Splint	Dynamic: moving parts • Flexor tendon repair splint • Extensor tendon repair splint • Radial palsy splint Volar splint Dorsal splint		4. Functional position 5. Therapeutic: strengthen weak muscle	
Brace	Foot attachments, Leg braces, Knee joint, Pelvic band, Milwaukee Brace, Cervical collar, Trunk- hip- knee-ankle- foot	Surgical steel, aluminum, leather, plastic	Support the body, prevent and correct deformity; control involuntary movements	Scoliosis Spinal cord injury Orthopedic deformities CP
Wheelchair, patient vehicles, tricycles, and scooters	Manual Battery powered Scooter: battery Folding	Light chromium plated, plastic, fabric, battery	Transport • Indoor • outdoor • transfer to car	Spinal cord injury Amputee Muscular dystrophy Multiple sclerosis Cerebral palsy

Category of Device	Types	Materials	Purpose	Disability Examples
Automobile controls	Upper extremity: hand controls Lower extremity controls	Metal, leather, plastic	Enable individuals with disabilities to drive Controls gas, brake, signals, dimmer switch, steering, and transmission	Amputee Spinal cord injury Traumatic brain injury Cerebral palsy
Slings	• Overhead (wheelchair) • Universal hemiplegic sling	Cotton webbing	Back support, flail shoulder, support subluxated shoulder joint	Quadriplegia Hemiplegia
Traction	Cervical, lumbar, pelvic	Cotton	Reduce pain by relieving pressure on joint	Dislocation, arthritis, herniated disc
Foot and shoe orthoses	Inserts, heel, cushions, sole vamps, pads	Leather, plastic, metal, cotton, sponge	Assist gait, reduce pain, correct deformity	Back pain, arthritis, hammer toes, leg shortening, cerebral palsy

(continued)

Table of Muscles

Muscles of the Back

Superficial Muscles

Muscles	Origin	Insertion	Innervation	Action
Trapezius	External occipital protuberance, superior nucal line, ligamentum nuchae, spines of C7–T12	Spine of scapula, acromion, and lateral third of clavicle	Spinal accessory n., C3–C4	Adducts, rotates, elevates, and depresses scapula
Levator scapulae	Transverse processes of C1–C4	Medial border of scapula	Nerves to levator scapulae, C3–C4; dorsal scapular n.	Elevates scapula
Rhomboid minor	Spines of C7–T1	Root of spine of scapula	Dorsal scapular n, C5	Adducts scapula
Rhomboid major	Spines of T2–T5	Medial border of scapula	Dorsal scapular n.	Adducts scapula
Latissimus dorsi	Spines of T5–T12, thoracodorsal fascia, iliac crest, ribs 9–12	Floor of bicipital groove of humerus	Thoracodorsal n.	Adducts, extends, and rotates arm medially

Muscles	Origin	Insertion	Innervation	Action
Intermediate Muscles				
Serratus posterior–superior	Ligamentum nuchae, supraspinal ligament, and spines of C7–T3	Upper border of ribs 2–5	Intercostal n., T1–T4	Elevates ribs
Serratus posterior–inferior	Supraspinous ligament and spines of T11–L3	Lower border of ribs 9–12	Intercostal n., T9–T12	Depresses ribs
Deep Muscles (Intrinsics)				
Superficial Layer of Deep Muscles (Spinotransverse Group)				
Splenius capitis	Inferior half of ligamentum nuchae, spinous processes of T1–T6	Lateral aspect of mastoid process, lateral third of superior nuchal line	Dorsal rami of inferior cervical n.	Alone, it laterally flexes and rotates head and neck to same side; it works with the other splenius muscle, to extend the head and neck
Splenius cervicis	Inferior half of ligamentum nuchae, spinous processes of T1–T6	Posterior tubercles of transverse processes of C1–C4	Dorsal rami of inferior cervical n.	Alone, it laterally flexes and rotates head and neck to same side; it works with the other splenius muscle, to extend the head and neck

(continued)

(continued)

Intermediate Layer of Deep Muscles (Sacrospinalis or Erector Spinae Group)

Muscles	Origin	Insertion	Innervation	Action
Iliocostalis (Lateral column)	Posterior part of iliac crest, posterior aspect of sacrum, sacroiliac ligaments, and sacral and inferior lumbar spinous processes	Angles of the ribs, cervical transverse processes	Dorsal rami of spinal n.	Bilaterally, they extend the head and vertebral column; unilaterally, they laterally flex the head or vertebral column
Longissimus (Intermediate column)	Posterior part of iliac crest, posterior aspect of sacrum, sacroiliac ligaments, and sacral and inferior lumbar spinous processes	Transverse processes of thoracic and cervical vertebrae, mastoid process	Dorsal rami of spinal n.	Same as above; also, the longissimus capitis rotates the head to the same side
Spinalis (Medial column)	Posterior part of iliac crest, posterior aspect of sacrum, sacroiliac ligaments, and sacral and inferior lumbar spinous processes	Spinous processes from lumbar to thoracic region	Dorsal rami of spinal n.	Bilaterally, they extend the head and vertebral column; unilaterally, they laterally flex the head or vertebral column

Muscles	Origin	Insertion	Innervation	Action
Deep Layer of Deep Muscles (Transversospinalis Group)				
Semispinalis thoracis	Transverse processes	Thoracic and cervical spinous processes	Dorsal rami of cervical spinal n.	Bilaterally, extends the cervical and thoracic regions of vertebral column; unilaterally, rotates toward the opposite side
Semispinalis cervicis	Transverse processes	Thoracic and cervical spinous processes	Dorsal rami of cervical spinal n.	Bilaterally, extends the cervical and thoracic regions of vertebral column; unilaterally, rotates toward the opposite side
Semispinalis capitis	Transverse processes of T1–T6	Medial half of area between superior and inferior nuchal line on occipital bone	Dorsal rami of cervical spinal n.	Bilaterally, extend the head; unilaterally, rotates toward the opposite side

(continued)

(continued)

Muscles	Origin	Insertion	Innervation	Action
Multifidus	Laminae of S4–C2	Span 1–3 vertebrae before inserting in spinous processes	Dorsal rami of cervical spinal n.	Bilaterally, extend the trunk and stabilize the vertebral column; unilaterally, flex the trunk laterally and rotate it to the opposite side
Rotators	Transverse processes	Base of the spinous process superior to vertebra of origin	Dorsal rami of cervical spinal n.	Rotate the superior vertebra to the opposite side and stabilize it
Segmental Muscles				
Interspinales	Spinous processes	Adjacent spinous processes	Dorsal rami of cervical spinal n.	Extend the vertebral column
Intertransversarii	Transverse processes	Adjacent transverse processes	Ventral and dorsal rami of cervical spinal n.	Bilaterally, extend the vertebral column; unilaterally, laterally flex the superior vertebra
Levator costarum	Transverse processes	Rib just inferior to vertebra of origin	Dorsal rami of spinal n.	Elevate the ribs during inspiration

Muscles	Origin	Insertion	Innervation	Action
Suboccipital Muscles				
Rectus capitis posterior major	Spine of axis	Lateral portion of inferior nuchal line	Suboccipital n.	Extends, rotates, and flexes head laterally
Rectus capitis posterior minor	Posterior tubercle of atlas	Occipital bone below inferior nuchal line	Suboccipital n.	Extends and flexes head laterally
Obliquus capitis superior	Transverse process of atlas	Occipital bone above inferior nuchal line	Suboccipital n.	Extends, rotates, and flexes head laterally
Obliquus capitis inferior	Spine of axis	Transverse process of atlas	Suboccipital n.	Extends head and rotates it laterally
Muscles of the Neck				
Platysma	Superficial fascia over upper part of deltoid and pectoralis major	Mandible; skin and muscles over mandible and angle of mouth	Facial n.	Depresses lower jaw and lip and angle of mouth; wrinkle skin of neck
Sternocleidomastoid	Manubrium sterni and medial one-third of clavicle	Mastoid process and lateral one-half of superior nuchal line	Spinal accessory n.; C2–C3 (sensory)	Unilaterally, turns face toward opposite side; bilaterally, flexes head, raises thorax

(continued)

Muscles	Origin	Insertion	Innervation	Action
Suprahyoid Muscles				
Digastric	Anterior belly from digstric fossa of mandible; posterior belly from mastoid notch	Intermediate tendon attached to body of hyoid	Anterior belly by mylohyoid n. of trigeminal n.; posterior belly by facial n.	Elevates hyoid and tongue; depresses mandible
Mylohyoid	Mylohyoid line of mandible	Median raphe and body of hyoid bone	Mylohyoid n. of trigeminal n.	Elevates hyoid and tongue; depresses mandible
Stylohyoid	Styloid process	Body of hyoid	Facial n.	Elevates hyoid
Geniohyoid	Genial tubercle of mandible	Body of hyoid	C1 via hypoglossal n.	Elevates hyoid and tongue
Infrahyoid Muscles				
Sternohyoid	Manubrium sterni and medial end of clavicle	Body of hyoid	Ansa cervicalis	Depresses hyoid and larynx
Sternothyroid	Manubrium sterni; first costal cartilage	Oblique line of thyroid cartilage	Ansa cervicalis	Depresses thyroid cartilage and larynx
Thyrohyoid	Oblique line of thyroid cartilage	Body and greater horn of hyoid	C1 via hypoglossal n.	Depresses and retracts hyoid and larynx

Muscles	Origin	Insertion	Innervation	Action
Omohyoid	Inferior belly from medial lip of suprascapular notch and suprascapular ligament; superior belly from intermediate tendon	Inferior belly to intermediate tendon; superior belly to body of hyoid	Ansa cervicalis	Depresses and retracts hyoid and larynx
Prevertebral Muscles				
Anterior scalene	Transverse processes of C3–C6	Scalene tubercle on first rib	Ventral rami of cervical spinal n. (C3–C8)	Elevates first rib, bends neck
Middle scalene	Transverse processes of C2–C7	Upper surface of first rib	Ventral rami of cervical spinal n. (C3–C8)	Flexes neck laterally, elevates first rib during forced inspiration
Posterior scalene	Transverse processes of C4–C6	Outer surface of second rib	Ventral rami of cervical spinal n. (C7–C8)	Flexes neck laterally, elevates second rib during forced inspiration
Longus capitis	Transverse processes of C3–C6	Basilar part of occipital bone	Ventral rami of cervical spinal n. (C1–C4)	Flexes and rotates head

(continued)

(continued)

Muscles	Origin	Insertion	Innervation	Action
Longus colli	Transverse processes and bodies of C3–T3	Anterior tubercle of atlas; bodies of C2–C4; transverse process of C5–C6	Ventral rami of cervical spinal n. (C2–C6)	Flexes and rotates head
Rectus capitis anterior	Lateral mass of atlas	Basilar part of occipital bone	Ventral rami of cervical spinal n. (C1–C2)	Flexes and rotates head
Rectus capitis lateralis	Transverse process of atlas	Jugular process of occipital bone	Ventral rami of cervical spinal n. (C1–C2)	Flexes head laterally
Muscles of Facial Expression				
Occipitofrontalis	Superior nuchal line; upper orbital margin	Epicranial aponeurosis	Facial n.	Elevates eyebrows, wrinkles forehead
Corrugator supercilii	Medial supraorbital margin	Skin of medial eyebrow	Facial n.	Draws eyebrows downward medially
Orbicularis oculi	Medial orbital margin; medial palpebral ligament; lacrimal bone	Skin and rim of orbit; tarsal plate; lateral palpebral raphe	Facial n.	Closes eyelids
Procerus	Nasal bone and cartilage	Skin between eyebrows	Facial n.	Wrinkles skin over bones

Muscles	Origin	Insertion	Innervation	Action
Nasalis	Maxilla lateral to incisive fossa	Ala of nose	Facial n.	Draws ala of nose toward septum
Depressor septi	Incisive fossa of maxilla	Ala and nasal septum	Facial n.	Constricts nares
Orbicularis oris	Maxilla above incisor teeth	Skin of lip	Facial n.	Closes lips
Levator anguli oris	Canine fossa of maxilla	Angle of mouth	Facial n.	Elevates angle of mouth meidally
Levator labii superioris	Maxilla above infraorbital foramen	Skin of upper lip	Facial n.	Elevates upper lip, dilates nares
Levator labii superioris alaeque nasi	Frontal process of maxilla	Skin of upper lip	Facial n.	Elevates ala of nose and upper lip
Zygomaticus major	Zygomatic arch	Angle of mouth	Facial n.	Draws angle of mouth backward and upward
Zygomaticus minor	Zygomatic arch	Angle of mouth	Facial n.	Elevates upper lip
Depressor labii inferioris	Mandible below mental foramen	Orbicularis oris and skin of lower lip	Facial n.	Depresses lower lip
Depressor anguli oris	Oblique line of mandible	Angle of mouth	Facial n.	Depresses angle of mouth
Risorius	Fascia over masseter	Angle of mouth	Facial n.	Retracts angle of mouth

(continued)

Muscles	Origin	Insertion	Innervation	Action
Buccinator	Mandible; pterygomandibular raphe; alveolar processes	Angle of mouth	Facial n.	Presses cheek to keep it taut
Mentalis	Incisive fossa of mandible	Skin of chin	Facial n.	Elevates and protrudes lower lip
Auricularis anterior, superior, and posterior	Temporal fascia; epicranial aponeurosis; mastoid process	Anterior, superior, and posterior sides of auricle	Facial n.	Retract and elevate ear
Muscles of Mastication				
Temporalis	Temporal fossa	Coronoid process and ramus of mandible	Trigeminal n.	Elevates and retracts mandible
Masseter	Lower border and medial surface of zygomatic arch	Lateral surface of coronoid process, ramus and angle of mandible	Trigeminal n.	Elevates mandible
Lateral pterygoid	Superior head from infratemporal surface of sphenoid; inferior head from lateral surface of lateral pterygoid plate	Neck of mandible; articular disk and capsule of temporomandibular joint	Trigeminal n.	Protracts (protrudes) and depresses mandible

Muscles	Origin	Insertion	Innervation	Action
Medial pterygoid	Tuber of maxilla; medial surface of lateral pterygoid plate; pyramidal process of palatine bone	Medial surface of angle and ramus of mandible	Trigeminal n.	Protracts (protrudes) and elevates mandible

Muscles of Eye Movement

Muscles	Origin	Insertion	Innervation	Action
Superior rectus	Common tendinous ring	Sclera just behind cornea	Oculomotor n.	Elevates eyeball
Inferior rectus	Same as above	Sclera just behind cornea	Oculomotor n.	Depresses eyeball
Medial rectus	Same as above	Sclera just behind cornea	Oculomotor n.	Adducts eyeball
Lateral rectus	Same as above	Sclera just behind cornea	Abducens n.	Adducts eyeball
Levator palpebrae superioris	Lesser wing of sphenoid above and anterior to optic canal	Tarsal plate and skin of upper eyelid	Oculomotor n.	Elevates upper eyelid
Superior oblique	Body of sphenoid bone above optic canal	Sclera beneath superior rectus	Trochlear n.	Rotates downward and medially, depresses adducted eye

(continued)

Muscles	Origin	Insertion	Innervation	Action
Inferior oblique	Floor of orbit lateral to lacrimal groove	Sclera beneath lateral rectus	Oculomotor n.	Rotates upward and laterally, elevates adducted eye
Muscles of the Palate				
Tensor veli palatini	Scaphoid fossa; spine of sphenoid; cartilage of auditory tube	Tendon hooks around hamulus of medial pterygoid plate to insert into aponeurosis of soft palate	Mandibular branch of trigeminal n.	Tenses soft palate
Levator veli palatini	Petrous part of temporal bone; cartilage of auditory tube	Aponeurosis of soft palate	Vagus n. via pharyngeal plexus	Elevates soft palate
Palatoglossus	Aponeurosis of soft palate	Dorsolateral side of tongue	Vagus n. via pharyngeal plexus	Elevates tongue
Palatopharyngeus	Aponeurosis of soft palate; hard palate	Thyroid cartilage and side of pharynx; muscles of pharynx	Vagus n. via pharyngeal plexus	Elevates pharynx; closes nasopharynx
Musculus uvulae	Posterior nasal spine of palatine bone; palatein aponeurosis	Mucous membrane of uvula	Vagus n. via pharyngeal plexus	Elevates uvula

Muscles	Origin	Insertion	Innervation	Action
Muscles of the Tongue				
Styloglossus	Styloid process	Side and inferior aspect of tongue	Hypoglossal n.	Retracts and elevates tongue
Hyoglossus	Body and greater horn of hyoid bone	Side and inferior aspect of tongue	Hypoglossal n.	Depresses and retracts tongue
Genioglossus	Genial tubercle of mandible	Inferior aspect of tongue; body of hyoid bone	Hypoglossal n.	Protrudes and depresses tongue
See Palatoglossus				
Muscles of the Pharynx				
Superior constrictor	Medial pterygoid plate; pterygoid hamulus; pterygo-mandibular raphe; mylohyoid line of mandible; side of tongue	Median raphe and pharyngeal tubercle of skull	Vagus n. via pharyngeal plexus	Constricts upper pharynx
Middle constrictor	Greater and lesser horns of hyoid; stylohyoid ligament	Median raphe	Vagus n. via pharyngeal plexus	Constricts lower pharynx
Inferior constrictor	Arch of cricoid and oblique line of thyroid cartilages	Median raphe of pharynx	Vagus n. via pharyngeal plexus, recurrent and external laryngeal n.	Constricts lower pharynx

(continued)

(continued)

Muscles	Origin	Insertion	Innervation	Action
Stylopharyngeus	Styloid process	Thyroid cartilage and muscles of pharynx	Glossopharyngeal n.	Elevates pharynx and larynx
Salpingopharyngeus	Cartilage of auditory tube	Muscles of pharynx	Vagus n. via pharyngeal plexus	Elevates nasopharynx, opens auditory tube
See Palatopharyngeus				
Muscles of the Larynx				
Cricothyroid	Arch of cricoid cartilage	Inferior horn and lower lamina of thyroid cartilage	External laryngeal n.	Tenses vocal folds
Posterior cricoarytenoid	Posterior surface of lamina of cricoid cartilage	Muscular process of arytenoid cartilage	Recurrent laryngeal n.	Abducts vocal folds
Lateral cricoarytenoid	Arch of cricoid cartilage	Muscular process of arytenoid cartilage	Recurrent laryngeal n.	Abducts vocal folds
Transverse arytenoid	Posterior surface of arytenoid cartilage	Opposite arytenoid cartilage	Recurrent laryngeal n.	Abducts vocal folds
Oblique arytenoid	Muscular process of arytenoid cartilage	Apex of opposite arytenoid	Recurrent laryngeal n.	Abducts vocal folds
Aryepiglottic	Apex of arytenoid cartilage	Side of epiglottic cartilage	Recurrent laryngeal n.	Abducts vocal folds

Muscles	Origin	Insertion	Innervation	Action
Thyroarytenoid	Inner surface of thyroid lamina	Lateral margin of epiglottic cartilage	Recurrent laryngeal n.	Adducts vocal folds
Thyroepiglottic	Anteromedial surface of lamina of thyroid cartilage	Vocal process	Recurrent laryngeal n.	Adducts and tenses vocal folds
Vocalis	Anteromedial surface of lamina of thyroid cartilage	Anterolateral surface of arytenoid cartilage	Recurrent laryngeal n.	Adducts vocal folds
Muscles of the Middle Ear				
Stapedius	Pyramidal eminence	Neck of the stapes	Branch of the facial n.	Pulls the head of the stapes posteriorly, thereby tilting the base of the stapes and protects the inner ear from injury during a loud noise
Tensor tympani	Cartilaginous portion of the auditory tube	Handle of the malleus	Mandibular branch of trigeminal n.	Draws the manubrium medially, pulling the tympanic membrane taut

(continued)

(continued)

Muscles	Origin	Insertion	Innervation	Action
Muscles of the Upper Limb				
Muscles of the Shoulder Region				
Deltoid	Lateral third of clavicle, acromion, and spine of scapula	Deltoid tuberosity of humerus	Axillary n.	Anterior part: flexes and medially rotates arm; Middle part: abducts arm; Posterior part: extends and laterally rotates arm
Supraspinatus	Supraspinous fossa of scapula	Superior facet of greater tubercle of humerus	Suprascapular n.	Abducts arm
Infraspinatus	Infraspinous fossa	Middle facet of greater tubercle of humerus	Suprascapular n.	Rotates arm laterally
Subscapularis	Subscapular fossa	Lesser tubercle of humerus	Upper and lower subscapular n.	Rotates arm medially
Teres Major	Dorsal surface of inferior angle of scapula	Medial lip of intertubercular groove of humerus	Lower subscapular n.	Adducts and rotates arm medially
Teres Minor	Upper portion of lateral border of scapula	Lower facet of greater tubercle of humerus	Axillary n.	Rotates arm laterally

Muscles	Origin	Insertion	Innervation	Action
Latissimus Dorsi	Spines of T7–T12 thoracolumbar fascia, iliac crest, ribs 9–12	Floor of bicipital groove of humerus	Thoracodorsal n.	Adducts, extends, and rotates arm medially
Muscles of the Arm				
Coracobrachialis	Coracoid process	Middle third of medial surface of humerus	Musculocutaneous n.	Flexes and adducts arm
Biceps Brachii	Long head: supraglenoid tubercle of scapula; short head: tip of coraciod process of scapula	Radial tuberosity of radius	Musculocutaneous n.	Flexes arm and forearm, supinates forearm when it is supine
Brachialis	Distal half of anterior surface of humerus	Coronoid process of ulna and ulnar tuberosity	Musculocutaneous n.	Flexes forearm
Triceps Brachii	Long head: infragenniod tubercle of scapula; Lateral head: posterior surface of humerus, superior to radial groove; Medial head: posterior surface of humerus, inferior radial groove	Posterior surface of olecranon process of ulna	Radial n.	Extends forearm

(continued)

(*continued*)

Muscles	Origin	Insertion	Innervation	Action
Anconeus	Lateral epicondyle of humerus	Olecranon and upper posterior surface of ulna	Radial n.	Extends forearm with triceps; stabilizes elbow joint
Muscles of the Anterior Forearm				
Pronator Teres	Medial epicondyle and coronoid process of ulna	Middle of lateral side of radius	Median n.	Pronates forearm
Flexor Carpi Radialis	Medial epicondyle of humerus	Bases of second and third metacarpals	Median n.	Flexes forearm, flexes and abducts hand
Palmaris Longus	Medial epicondyle of humerus	Flexor retinaculum, palmar aponeurosis	Median n.	Flexes hand and forearm
Flexor Carpi Ulnaris	Medial epicondyle, medial olecranon, and posterior border of ulna	Pisiform, hook of hamate, and base of fifth metacarpal	Ulnar n.	Flexes and adducts hand, flexes forearm
Flexor Digitorum Superficialis	Medial epicondyle, coronoid process, oblique line of radius	Middle phalanges of finger	Median n.	Flexes proximal interphalangeal joints, flexes hand and forearm
Flexor Digitorum Profundus	Anteromedial surface of ulna, interosseous membrane	Bases of distal phalanges of fingers	Ulnar and median n.	Flexes distal interphalangeal joints and hand

Muscles	Origin	Insertion	Innervation	Action
Flexor Pollicis Longus	Anterior surface of radius, interosseous membrane, and coronoid process	Base of distal phalanx of thumb	Median n.	Flexes thumb
Pronator Quadratus	Anterior surface of dital ulna	Anterior surface of distal radius	Median n.	Pronates forearm
Muscles of the Posterior Forearm				
Brachioradialis	Lateral supracondylar ridge of humerus	Base of radial styloid process	Radial n.	Flexes forearm
Extensor Carpi Radilais Longus	Lateral supracondllar ridge of humerus	Dorsum of base of second metacarpal	Radial n.	Extends and abducts hand
Extensor Carpi Radialis Brevis	Lateral epicondyle of humerus	Posterior base of third metacarpal	Radial n.	Extends fingers and abducts hands
Extensor Digitorum	Lateral epicondyle of humerus	Extensor expansion, base of middle and digital phalanges	Radial n.	Extends fingers and hand
Extensor Digiti Minimi	Common extensor tendon and interosseoue membrane	Extensor expansion, base of middle and distal phalanges	Radial n.	Extends little finger
Extensor Carpi Ulnaris	Lateral epicondyle and posterior surface of ulna	Base of fifth	Radial n.	Extends and adducts hand

(continued)

Muscles	Origin	Insertion	Innervation	Action
Supinator	Lateral epicondyle, radial collateral ad anular ligaments	Lateral side of upper part of radius	Radial n.	Supinates forearm
Abductor Pollicis Longus	Interosseous membrane, middle third of posterior surfaces of radius and ulna	Lateral surface of base of first metacarpal	Radial n.	Abducts thumb and hand
Extensor Pollicis Longus	Interosseous membrane and middle third of posterior surface of ulna	Base of distal phalanx of thumb	Radial n.	Extends distal phalanx of thumb and abducts hand
Extensor Pollicis Brevis	Interosseous membrane and posterior surface of middle third radius	Base of proximal phalanx of thumb	Radial n.	FExtends proximal phlanx of thumb and abducts hand
Extensor Indicis	Posterior surface of ulna and interosseous membrane	Extensor expansion of index finger	Radial n.	Extneds index finger
Muscles of the Hand				
Abductor Pollicis Brevis	Flexor retinaculum, scaphoid, and trapezium	Lateral side of base of proximal phalanx of thumb	Median n.	Abducts thumb

Muscles	Origin	Insertion	Innervation	Action
Flexor Pollicis Brevis	Flexor retinaculum and trapezium	Base of proximal phalanx of thumb	Median n.	Flexes thumb\
Opponens Pollicis	Flexor retinaculum and trapezium	Lateral side of first metacarpal	Median n.	Opposes thumb to other digits
Adductor pollicis	Oblique head: capitate and bases of second and third metacarpals; Transverse head: palmar surface of third metacarpal	Medial side of base of proximal phalanx of thumb	Ulnar n.	Adducts thumb
Palmaris Brevis	Medial side of flexor retinaculum, palmar aponeurosis	Skin of medial side of palm	Ulnar n.	Wrinkles skin on medial side of palm
Abductor Digiti Minimi	Pisiform and tendon of flexor carpi ulanris	Medial side of base of proximal phalanx of little finger	Ulnar n.	Abducts little finger
Flexor Digiti Minimi Brevis	Flexor retinaculum and hook of hamate	Medial side of base of proximal phalanx of little finger	Ulnar n.	Flexes proximal phalanx of little finger
Opponens Digiti Minimi	Flexor retinaculum and hook of hamate	Medial side of fifth metacarpal	Ulnar n.	Opposes little finger

(continued)

(continued)

Muscles	Origin	Insertion	Innervation	Action
Lumbricals (4)	Lateral side of tendons of flexor digitorum profundus	Lateral side of extensor expansion	Median (2 lateral) and ulnar (2 medial) n.	Flex metacarpophalangeal joints and extend interphalangeal joints
Dorsal interossei (4)	Adjacent sides of metacarpal bones	Lateral sides of bases of proximal phalanges; extensor expansion	Ulnar n.	Abduct fingers; flex metacarpophalangeal joints; extend interphalangeal joints
Palmar interossei (3)	Medial side of second metacarpal; lateral sides of fourth and fifth metacarpals	Bases of proximal phalanges in same sides as their origins; extensor expansion	Ulnar n.	Adduct fingers; flex metacarpophalangeal joints; extend interphalangeal joints

APPENDIX E

Average ROM Measurements

Shoulder

Flexion	0–180°
Extension	0–60°
Adduction/Abduction	0–180°
Horizontal Abduction	0–90°
Horizontal Adduction	0–45°
Internal Rotation	0–70°
External Rotation	0–90°
Internal Rotation (alternate method)	0–80°
External Rotation (alternate method)	0–60°

Elbow and Forearm

Extension/Flexion	0–150°
Supination	0–80°
Pronation	0–80°

Wrist

Flexion	0–80°
Extension	0–70°
Ulnar Deviation	0–30°
Radial Deviation	0–20°

Thumb

CM Flexion	0–15°
CM Extension	0–20°
MP Extension/Flexion	0–50°
IP Extension/Flexion	0–80°
Abduction	Cm
Opposition	Cm

Fingers

MP Flexion	0–90°
PIP Extension/Flexion	0–100°

DIP Extnesion/Flexion	0–90°
Abduction	No Norm
Adduction	No Norm

APPENDIX F

Prime Movers for Upper and Selected Lower Extremity Motions

Scapular elevation	Upper trapezius
	Levator scapulae
Scapular depression	Lower trapezius
	Latissimus dorsi
Scapular adduction	Middle trapezius
	Rhomboids
Scapular abduction	Serratus anterior
Shoulder flexion	Anterior deltoid
	Coracobrachialis
	Pectoralis major, clavicular head
	Biceps, both heads
Shoulder extension	Latissimus dorsi
	Teres major
	Posterior deltoid
	Triceps, long head
Shoulder abduction	Supraspinatus
	Middle deltoid
Shoulder adduction	Pectoralis major
	Teres major
	Latissimus dorsi
Shoulder horizontal abduction	Posterior deltoid
Shoulder horizonta adduction	Pectoralis major
	Anterior deltoid
Shoulder external rotation	Infraspinatus
	Teres minor
	Posterior deltoid
Shoulder internal rotation	Subscapularis
	Teres major
	Latissimus dorsi
	Pectoralis major
	Anterior deltoid

Elbow flexion	Biceps
	Brachialis
	Brachioradialis
Elbow extension	Triceps
Pronation	Pronator teres
	Pronator quadratus
Supination	Supinator
	Biceps
Wrist extension	Extensor carpi radialis longus (ECRL)
	Extensor carpi radialis brevis (ECRB)
	Extensor carpi ulnaris (ECU)
Wrist flexion	Flexor carpi radialis (FCR)
	Palmaris longus
	Flexor carpi ulnaris (FCU)
Finger DIP flexion	Flexor digitorum profundus (FDP)
Finger PIP flexion	Flexor digitorum superficialis (FDS)
	Flexor digitorum profundus (FDP)
Finger MP flexion	Flexor digitorum profundus (FDP)
	Flexor digitorum superficialis (FDS)
	Dorsal interossei
	Volar (palmar) interossei
	Flexor digiti minimi (small finger only)
Finger adduction	Volar (palmar) interossei
Finger abduction	Dorsal interossei
	Abductor digiti minimi (small finger only)

Finger MP extension	Extensor digitorum (ED)
	Extensor indicis proprius (index finger only)
	Extensor digiti minimi (small finger only)
Finger PIP/DIP extension	Lumbricales
	Dorsal and volar (palmar) interossei
	Extensor digitorum (ED)
	Extensor indicis proprius (index finger only)
	Extensor digiti minimi (small finger only)
Thumb IP extension	Extensor pollicis longus (EPL)
Thumb MP extension	Extensor pollicis brevis (EPB)
	Extensor pollicis longus (EPL)
Thumb abduction	Abductor pollicis longus (APL)
	Abductor pollicis brevis (APB)
Thumb IP flexion	Flexor pollicis longus (FPL)
Thumb MP flexion	Flexor pollicis brevis (FPB)
	Flexor pollicis longus (FPL)
Thumb adduction	Adductor pollicis
Opposition	Opponens pollicis (thumb)
	Opponens digiti minimi (small finger)
Hip flexion	Iliopsoas - Iliacus and psoas major
Hip extension	Gluteus maximus
	Biceps femoris
Knee flexion	Semimembranosus

	Semitendinosus
	Biceps femoris
Knee extension	Rectus femoris
	Vastus medialis
	Vastus intermedius
	Vastus lateralis
Ankle dorsiflexion	Tibialis anterior
	Extensor hallucis longus
	Extensor digitorum longus
Ankle plantar flexion	Gastrocnemius
	Soleus

APPENDIX G

Substitutions for Muscle Contraction

Scapular elevation	Pushing on the knees when sitting
Scapular depression	Gravity if sitting or using the fingers to inch the arm downward along a surface if prone
Scapular adduction	Gravity if sitting
Scapular abduction	Using the fingers to inch the arm outward along a surface if supine
Shoulder flexion	Trunk extension or substitution by shoulder abductors
Shoulder extension	Hunching the shoulders forward or shoulder abductors
Shoulder abduction	Long head of the biceps if humerus is externally rotated or trunk lateral flexion
Shoulder adduction	Gravity if sitting or using the fingers to inch the arm downward along a surface if supine
Shoulder horizontal abduction	Trunk rotation
Shoulder horizontal adduction	Trunk rotation
Shoulder external rotation	Scapula adduction + downward rotation, the triceps, or supination
Shoulder internal rotation	Scapula abduction + upward rotation, the triceps, or pronation
Elbow flexion	Wrist flexors

Elbow extension	Gravity if sitting or external rotation to help gravity assist if in gravity-eliminated position
Pronation	Wrist and finger flexors
Supination	Wrist and finger extensors
Wrist extension	Extensor pollicis longus, extensor digitorum
Wrist flexion	Abductor pollicis longus, flexor pollicis longus, flexor digitorum superficialis, and flexor digitorum profundus
Finger DIP flexion	Rebound of fingers following extension or tenodesis
Finger PIP flexion	Rebound of fingers following extension or tenodesis
Finger MP flexion	Rebound of fingers following extension or tenodesis
Finger adduction	Extrinsic finger flexors or gravity for first palmar interosseus
Finger abduction	Extensor digitorum or gravity for dorsal interossei 3 and 4 and abductor digiti minimi
Finger MP extension	Rebound of fingers following flexion or tenodesis
Finger PIP/DIP extension	Other muscles of extension if MP is flexed
Thumb IP extension	Rebound of thumb following flexion, abductor pollicis brevis, adductor pollicis, and flexor pollicis brevis
Thumb MP extension	Rebound of thumb following flexion
Thumb abduction	Extensor pollicis brevis

Thumb IP flexion	Rebound of thumb following extension
Thumb MP flexion	Rebound of thumb following extension, abductor pollicis brevis, and adductor pollicis
Thumb adduction	Extensor pollicis longus, flexor pollicis longus, and flexor pollicis brevis
Opposition	Abductor pollicis brevis, flexor pollicis brevis, and flexor pollicis longus